Vibrational Healing

Vibrational Healing

REVEALING THE ESSENCE OF NATURE

THROUGH

AROMATHERAPY'S USE OF ESSENTIAL OILS

DEBORAH EIDSON

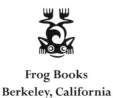

Frog Books
Berkeley, California

Published by Frog Books, an imprint of
North Atlantic Books
P.O. Box 12327
Berkeley, California 94712

Book cover and interior design by Carolina de Bartolo
Illustrations by Mykol Blackwell
Printed in the United States of America

Vibrational Healing: Revealing the Essence of Nature through Aromatherapy's Use of Essential Oils is sponsored by the Society for the Study of Native Arts and Sciences, a nonprofit educational corporation whose goals are to develop an educational and cross-cultural perspective linking various scientific, social, and artistic fields; to nurture a holistic view of arts, sciences, humanities, and healing; and to publish and distribute literature on the relationship of mind, body, and nature.

North Atlantic Books' publications are available through most bookstores. For further information, visit our website at www.northatlanticbooks.com or call 800-733-3000.

ISBN-13: 978-1-58394-031-0

Library of Congress Cataloging-in-Publication Data
        Eidson, Deborah, 1956–
                Vibrational healing : revealing the essence of nature through aromatherapy's use of essential oils / Deborah Eidson.
            p. cm.
        Includes bibliographical references.
        ISBN 1-58394-031-6 (alk. paper)
        1. Aromatherapy. 2. Vibration—Therapeutic use. I. Title.

        RM666.A68E38 2000
        615'.321—dc21
                                                                00-037652
                                                                CIP

3   4   5   6   7   8   9   SHERIDAN   17   16   15   14   13   12

Dedication

I dedicate this book to the memory of three special people who passed before its publication. I miss their physical presence but feel their Spiritual essence awakening me to a greater vision of existence.

To my Grandmother, Annie Caroon

Who instilled eccentricity
Who began my metaphysical training
Who opened the door to the realms of the unknown!
Thank You for blessing me with the gift for healing.

To my Mother, Victoria Eidson

Who helped to awaken my Soul's purpose
Who encouraged me to realize my dreams.
Thank you for making it all possible.

To my beloved friend and partner, Rex Howe

You shared with me the greatest gift of all.
It's stronger than death.
Our hearts still dance to the sacred tune of love,
Weaving a pattern of light bonding us together through eternity,
Evolving a bridge to cross the chasm of separation into oneness.
Ours Souls intertwined together forever—from life to the beyond.
Thank you for teaching me to love myself.

A special thanks to the many people who helped and encouraged me to write this book: all my clients who helped me experiment with the oils; my friends, Diane Roman and Erica Nelson, for their immense help reviewing and clarifying the information; and my Angel of an editor, Liz Davidson, and her talent for eloquent writing.

Contents

Preface

My intention in writing this book is to share techniques that empower and encourage an individual to develop a deeper relationship with Spirit. Vibrational aromatherapy provides a variety of tools for practitioners or lay people to use on themselves, clients, friends, and families in the birthing of their Spiritual Selves.

This book is a synthesis of my personal experiences of working with the essential oils on myself and on clients in my private practice for the last ten years. Through learning to work with the subtle energies and the essential oils in my practice, I have experienced first-hand how essential oils have activated positive changes in my life and the lives of others. The positive results I've achieved by using and interacting with the oils' energy are the instrumental reason I want to share this information. I draw upon my training and certifications in NLP, Time Line, Hypnosis, Touch for Health, Polarity, Massage, and Cranial-Sacral therapy, as well as with Aromatherapy. My training, along with my developed intuition and additional study of the historical, traditional, and vibratory uses of the oils, has influenced my conception of their physical, emotional, mental, and spiritual uses. This book assimilates and interprets information gathered over many years and consolidates it into techniques that are conducive to enhancing the oils' effects. The combined group effort of my friends, colleagues, clients, and the oils themselves has contributed to the manifestation of this book.

More than anything, this book is about spirituality, which is an individual's evolution towards a fulfilling, joyous love for self that allows Spirit to manifest. Spirituality is the journey to reunite with Source. The Spiritual path induces a strong healthy sense of inner worth that allows one to love and honor Self. This sense of worth, in turn, reflects out into the world as love, compassion and Grace. These are the energies that manifest when the Soul or Spirit integrates with the personality. It is living life based on principles of unconditional love for Self and humanity. To actualize unconditional love requires taking full responsibility for all actions and thoughts. Spirituality inspires an individual to become more conscious and present for living in the moment.

You are responsible for the life that you live, and if it is not a nourishing environment for your Soul's purpose you will always feel a yearning for something unidentified. To discover what is missing, act upon the restlessness as an invitation to embark on a pilgrimage. This journey could better acquaint you with your true self, or Spirit. Discovering your spirituality results in the integration of your personality with Spirit, thus creating a vehicle for manifesting Spirit on this physical plane.

The spiritual journey will lead you to the darkest regions of your soul in order to liberate you from fear. This will be the most challenging and thrilling adventure you will ever have. The experience will have moments of pure bliss coupled with times of immense pain and suffering that will test your faith and desire for this union. The toll exacted on this road of change can feel quite exorbitant because it demands total honesty with your self, total commitment to your path, as well as perseverance towards your goal.

The key to walking the spiritual path is recognizing, accepting, and making friends with your shadow-self. There will be times when the resistance and revulsion will seem so overwhelming and you will become discouraged. It is natural for you to question the sanity of this quest, as well as wonder if it is worth the effort to endure this journey. It will feel at times that it is easier to live in your pain than make the change to continue the pursuit. At this time, the tendency to rationalize arises. You might try to convince yourself that your life is fine and there is no real reason to push you onward. Beware that you are being seduced to stay in your rut. Rationalization is one of the greatest obstacles, because it justifies the creation and maintenance of illusions that distort perception. It takes immense courage to see your reality in the truth of Spirit.

We are masters of creating distractions that divert us from discovering our purpose. Mass culture has sold us the illusion of the quick fix, but true change only comes from a focused intention to reprogram our entrenched habits and beliefs. We must understand the magnetic force that our words, thoughts, and deeds generate. Being responsible for ourselves allows us to truly reclaim our power and create the life we want.

The benefit of undergoing the arduous journey of self-discovery is a grander picture of life. Comprehension of the greater design of life begins to dawn in you. You are liberated from limitation, and all becomes possible. Abundance replaces lack and destitution. Loneliness, depression, and worries are diminished through the love and compassion of Spirit. The greatest gift of all is an enriched sense of wonder and joy. You begin attuning to the heartbeat of oneness and the miracle of life's diversity. The currents of Spirit run through you, and direct you towards experiencing the perfection of existence.

It is important to keep this book in perspective. It is not intended to replace the services of medical or psychological treatment when needed, and this book is not meant to be your only tool. It is important to use this information in combination with other growth and healing processes such as counseling and therapy, self-help groups, support groups, and health care. Use any traditional or alternative healing methods that generate a holistic integration of your body, mind, and spirit. My intention is to inform and provide tools with which to stimulate greater awareness and understanding, as well as activate the desire in you to take an active part in your healing process. As with all things, do not blindly adhere to this information. If it works for you, then use it. If it does not ring true for you, then let it go. It is more important to honor your truth.

I have developed a unique relationship with each oil. I recognize them as teachers as well as the light consciousness known as Devic beings. The oils are a gift from the Plant Kingdom and are a bridge by which to interact with them. Since I recognize them as teachers, I capitalize their names. I hope that you, too, will cross that bridge and delight in the wondrous life force of Unconditional Love and great joy they want to impart to us. The Devic energies of the Plant Kingdom will appear in your life if you maintain an open mind and have a desire to communicate with them. It is essential that you invite their presence and welcome their contribution. They could give you a gift that might appear as a wispy scent, a whisper on the wind, or a demonstration of the immense life force they embody. They might show themselves to you in meditation, dreams, visions, and intuitive flashes. Sometimes you will experience a wondrous feeling of love and become filled with bliss and total acceptance for the perfection of being exactly who and what you are.

Consequently, a desire will overcome and inspire you to spend more time in nature. You will feel an increased awe and wonderment with life. Encounters with the Devas will further heighten your skills for observing each plant's individual characteristics, signature, and beauty. This awakens in you a form of telepathy between the realms. Butterflies, bees, dragonflies, hummingbirds, lizards, and other creatures become attracted to your environment. By observing and meditating on their presence you invite them into your life, and you will receive messages helping you on the path. You will begin to understand the true language of life, and along with that will be greater guidance, assurance, and encouragement to walk your path with joy.

With each step we take closer to nature, we are rewarded with numerous gifts. Attuning with nature can help to reestablish our natural rhythms with the earth, enhancing our will to live, filling us with spiritual purpose and a blissful inner-peace. A deeper understanding will lead us to our foreordained role as Co-Creators and to become energy conductors manifesting and anchoring spiritual energy on this plane. Our transformation will influence everything that surrounds us, and it will assist in building new foundations for realities created with love and respect for this planet and most of all for ourselves and each other. We help Gaia advance on her path of evolution and the restoration of Eden. Healing ourselves raises the consciousness of our families, friends, and society. Honoring the life force in everything, we relearn how to walk upon the Earth more gently and reverently.

I am greatly humbled by all the teachers and challenges in my life that have promoted my Spiritual growth and my ability to enthusiastically celebrate life. The process of writing this book has been the most wondrous opportunity for me to surface, address, and resolve issues that have been unconsciously directing my life. This experience has also heightened my innate intuitive abilities, making me multi-sensory. Furthermore, it has ignited my Spiritual purpose and instigated an extraordinary amount of joy and an extraordinary inner-peace that I have never known. I have glimpsed a possible future of a magnificent journey propelling humanity into an unlimited state of abundance.

I thank all the Beings of Light that have worked with me, through me, and as me to accomplish this task. I ask for their continued support and direction in my life and yours—if you desire, invite their presence and be open to receive them.

I dedicate this book to people who are making a conscious decision to change their lives by taking responsibility for their healing process. The spiritual path will lead you to a more joyous life.

—Deborah Eidson
Light Worker for the New Millennium

Vibrational Healing
& Aromatherapy

Vibrational aromatherapy is a method of healing your physical, emotional, mental, and spiritual bodies using the energetic properties of essential oils. This healing process realizes a love of Self and a love of others that inspires spiritual growth.

Vibrational aromatherapy provides a means of co-creating with the Plant Kingdom to perceive and manifest an expanded reality. The essential oils help to stimulate energetic states of consciousness that open new channels of awareness. Opening up to these states of consciousness can help you discover insights into the causes of personal suffering in this life, healing the traumas by learning their spiritual lessons. The effectiveness of vibrational aromatherapy is a result of your intention, effort, and desire to promote change in your life.

Making changes in your life requires courage and determination. The essential oils are energetic tools and catalysts for change. For instance, if you have a reoccurring pattern of behavior (a tendency to maintain certain reactions instead of making new choices) causing distress in your life, changing your perception of the pattern from a problem to an opportunity to grow helps overcome it. Essential oils can assist in an introspective investigation of the root causes of your reactions and help you recall the experience that originally created the pattern. You will learn to feel in your body how attached you are to emotions and patterns related to those root causes.

The energies of the oils will make you conscious of your emotional reactions and help you evaluate whether they are appropriate responses to what is actually happening or if they are automatic responses which signal that an unconscious fragment of your personality has taken control of your reality. This unconscious part could be formed by beliefs or decisions made early in your life, in the womb, in a past life, or that are genealogically inherited. This part manifests by constantly *re-acting* that decision or belief. The thoughts and actions that shape your reality are not choices based in the moment, but *re-actions*. Often the incidents that formed these beliefs or decisions were taken out of context. Erroneous childhood perceptions of not being loved, wanted, or deserving become deeply embedded in your psyche, limiting and sabotaging your self-esteem and spiritual growth. Finding these incidents requires searching through your unconscious and feeling the emotional charges you have attached to your behavior. Honestly acknowledging feelings and admitting to the decisions or beliefs that you made from that first experience is a step to resolving a pattern. Reviewing the incident from a different standpoint allows for surprising insights. Often you will discover that these challenges were instrumental in building character and have always served you in some way. You can then take responsibility for having chosen the lesson. Another insight to be gained is the understanding that other people involved were acting out a role in your drama, and were not the cause of your feelings or behavior. Realizing this promotes healing your relationships with others.

Acknowledging how old lessons served you allows you to choose whether to react in the same old way, or to choose a new path. An exercise discussed in the next chapter, "Embracing into Love," is a meditation process that lovingly confronts painful incidents and feelings by disengaging from their emotional charge, thus beginning the journey toward healing and wholeness.

The properties of different oils can help with a variety of energy blocks that limit your spiritual growth and health—harboring bitterness and resentment, blaming others for your experiences, holding on to or denying hurts and transgressions, becoming too involved in other people's dramas, not taking responsibility for nurturing yourself. Holding on only prolongs the pain and keeps the wound open and active. Your attitudes, convictions, beliefs, and judgments create your reality and you are responsible for the types of experiences you attract. True nurturing and replenishment of energy come from communion with Spirit.

It is important to be aware that using vibrational aromatherapy with a focused intent has the potential to uncover many memories, decisions, and beliefs that have root causes extending into childhood, the womb, or past-life experiences. It can help you recognize inherited genealogical patterns. These all influence the attitudes and the causes of your reactions in the present, especially when they are unresolved issues. This knowledge is consciously forgotten, but the unconscious remembers it and bases its reactions on it, particularly if the unconscious is working to repress and deny trauma. Recovery of repressed feelings and memories begins the process of detoxifying the physical, emotional, and mental bodies, often inducing the condition known as a healing crisis, which results in a greater sense of well being.

What is termed as a healing crisis is caused by the etheric, emotional, and mental bodies detoxifying faster than the physical body can release. The healing crisis can mimic the flu or activate an old injury that holds the energy of the issue you are working on. As these feelings or pain arise, realize that they originate in the past and are discharging from the body. Awareness of this will keep you from becoming overwhelmed by the emotions that enact old patterns. If you are unable to process the emotions and begin engaging in the old patterns, it is necessary to seek outside help to gain clarity. You need help to rise above the trees in order to see the forest.

It is extremely important not to become attached to the energies surfacing, but to disconnect by acknowledging them and their root cause. Be cautious not to justify them as being caused by a present situation. Frequently the present situation is only a trigger, not the true cause. Watch for an inclination to rationalize feelings. Rationalization only leads to repression or denial. Honor yourself by truthfully feeling the emotion. If it is necessary, cry, rage, scream, or write exactly how the experience has affected you. Do not deny your feelings by attempting to persuade yourself that you have forgiven the experience, or by telling yourself "spiritual people do not feel that way."

All emotions are Spiritual, and the most important thing to learn is to truthfully acknowledge how you feel. Honesty requires examining your fears by asking what is the worst thing that can happen if they were to come true. Then ask, how likely is that to occur? This can help you to rediscover the humor you have lost on the journey, because most fears are totally irrational, formed by some internal belief or imagined inadequacy. Train yourself to be aware of your emotions, and learn to stop and question whether they are a choice or a *re-action*.

This questioning is called discernment, and is not to be confused with judgment. Discernment is a choice of preference, whereas judgment disregards the value or merit of the experience. Being honest and present with your emotions expands the heart's capability to experience deeper feelings of love and compassion.

Understanding the inner lesson that created an experience arrives by taking responsibility for it and knowing that it served you in some way. This conception ends the need to re-experience it and restores the possibility for harmonious realities to become established in your life. This promotes the healing of any disease that is potentially manifesting on the etheric or is already present in the physical body. Always remember that you choose the lessons that enhance your spiritual growth.

The oils reawaken the memory of joy while also illuminating the obstacles that keep the Self in a state of separation from Source. They serve as a means to stimulate aspirations for embarking on the journey of self-discovery, leading you to accept full responsibility for your life and the creation of your reality. They also permit you to become open to the vast realm of possibilities, encouraging you to become empowered by your own personal truth.

Using the essential oils with a focused intent will help you to acknowledge and achieve liberation from the issue. Vibrational aromatherapy expands your conscious perception of subtle energies occurring above the range of the conscious consensual reality. You will receive assistance from the Unseen Realm by asking for it and affirming its existence. This help is always available but we have separated our selves from it because we have felt unworthy to ask for, or receive it. Know that help is available even in your darkest distress if you remember to call upon it and are open to receiving it.

Learning to listen and act upon your intuition will always provide solutions for your dilemmas. The key is being observant of these subtle perceptions and learning to trust and rely upon the information you receive. You will begin to realize that you are not here alone, there are many beings that are sending you love and encouragement to carry out your mission.

Vibrational aromatherapy heightens your awareness, develops telepathy, intuition, and increases extra-sensory abilities. This expanded awareness of energy also helps to open and develop channels of communication from other realms of Light Beings, Spirit Guides, and Nature Spirits. These realms can be catalysts that encourage intuition, knowing, and the ability to receive guidance from Spirit, enhancing the quality of your life by inducing harmony, balance, joy, and inner-peace. Your reception of this increased love or light into your being radiates and instills it into everything you do, effecting and anchoring more light upon the Earth plane. The spiritual growth you experience on your journey of self-discovery will light the path and can encourage others to embark upon their own spiritual quest.

Vibrational Theory

Light is pure Spirit, which is the substance from which all life emerges. Through the refraction of light various vibrational frequencies, known as the ethers, are created. All creation originates from the vibrations of the ethers. The ethers emit the energy that creates the matter existing in this dimension of time and space. This vibrating flow of energy is what connects all beings with all existence. This interweaving of energy creates the state of Oneness. Spirit is this state of oneness.

On this Earth plane the nature of creation is constrained by the physical laws of time and space. Matter is shaped, formed and bound together into density though the exertion and motion of two forces of energy, which are *positive* and *negative*. These forces cannot be judged as good or evil, because Spirit in its true unified form contains both energies in its neutral state of oneness. Separation comes about through resistance, which results in the division of energy into polarities.

Just as there are only two polarities of energy, accordingly there are only two emotions: *Love* and *Fear*. That which is not Love is Fear. The acts of judging, disregarding, or invalidating an emotion, thought, or experience create resistance and separate Spirit into the polarities. Emotions are currents of energy with different frequencies, containing different experiences and lessons. They act as a prism that fractures the personality, creating a multitude of colorful facets for experiencing life. Reuniting the shattered parts of the personality opens a channel to align with Spirit, thus creating the multi-faceted light body to radiate the rainbow of Love.

All matter radiates an energy that extends beyond the confines of the physical. This is known as the etheric body. Each etheric body generates wave patterns, which are influenced by thought, movement, magnetism, and electricity. All thoughts are a form of energy stimulating the vibrational patterns and creating manifestation. Wave forms come into resonance by attracting and bonding to similar substances harmonious to their frequency, while repulsing that which is not of the same frequency. For example, when you are in a calm and loving state, you will attract those high-frequency types of experiences, and people compatible to this frequency will come into your life. Accordingly, when you are in a negative, fear-based state, your life will experience a downward spiraling into density. Dwelling on fear engages the law of attraction and magnetizes those experiences to surround you. Unfortunately, it is easier to bond to fear because it is so much more prevalent than love. Correspondingly, the ethers are instrumental in channeling more light into a person bonded to the positive because they contain less resistance and are more open to receiving Love. It is easier for a positive person to achieve a state of wholeness because there is simply less resistance.

According to the law of attraction, whatever we concentrate on we manifest. As a result, whatever we fear we manifest because emotions are currents of energy. By the same token, whatever we invalidate has to be manifested in order for us to learn the lesson of that experience, as well as the value of its existence.

To restore Spirit into wholeness, all negative fear energy must be embraced into love without judgment. Once the energy is embraced there is no resistance or separation and we return to the state of wholeness. The Soul loves without judgment; it is only the personality that makes judgments. Embracing all experiences with love teaches Divine Allowance for all things, which increases the capacity to feel compassion for the choices and lessons of others and our Self. This leads to a state of non-judgment. Having preferences or inclinations towards a particular feeling or choice of experience does not invalidate its worthiness, but allows for making choices harmonious to energy. Balancing the polarities occurs by ultimately surrendering judgment into acceptance and allowance. Those particular experiences will no longer need to manifest.

The polluting effect of negative thoughts is an encumbering burden in a person's life and energy field. It is a significant factor in creating and maintaining etheric density. This density is not usually perceived on a conscious level and often feels quite natural. Negative thought patterns molded by fear are a cause of ill health in the body, mind, and emotions and weaken the spirit. Disease always begins on the etheric level before it affects the physical. When the Spirit is impoverished it creates an opportunity for disease to manifest. When you experience a taste of spiritual purpose, dense energy starts to feel very suffocating.

Becoming aware of your mind chatter is an insightful tool for truthfully perceiving yourself and that which you are attracting into your life. Truthful perceptions are instrumental for attracting more harmonious love-based thought forms. Understanding how beliefs and thoughts are instrumental in developing unhealthy patterns leads to the realization of the influential role they play in creating disease. It is crucial to surface, acknowledge, and embrace repressed and fearful emotions to initiate the healing process of a disease or the potential of disease.

Discovering the need to experience disease and how it serves you is another key in the healing process. The body has a template encoded with the knowledge of perfect physical health. Resolving the resistance that distorts this information opens the template for restoring physical health.

Vibrational Healing

Vibrational healing is powerful and encompassing because it is not encumbered with the restrictions of time and space. Healing on a vibrational level is possible because all time is *Now*. In truth, there are no barriers of time and space. We call this expanded perception of reality the time-space continuum.

Our third dimensional reality is one of linear time. This is how the human brain orders its memories, so that it knows the difference between the past, present and future. Time is only a thought. We have amassed a reality based upon a subjective mechanical measurement of time that is totally out of rhythm with our own innate cycles. Understanding the true essence of time restores harmony. In the greater continuum of time and space, *Now* is simultaneously the past, present, and future. Learning to step out of this dimension comes by incorporating the time-space continuum into your life, which will diminish the control that mechanical time has over your life.

To understand the time-space continuum, consider that every choice you make or contemplate has many probable effects. Consciously training your intent to accept unlimited possibility stimulates your ability to perceive different dimensions. Opening and expanding your third eye helps you become acquainted with and receptive to information received from other dimensions. You can develop an innate talent for understanding and interpreting the information communicated and encoded in various forms of symbolic representation. This leads to comprehending what it means to be multi-dimensional.

To understand the time-space continuum, visualize yourself standing on a high mountain, with a view of the entire realm of possibilities. Imagine seeing lines of energy radiating out from your body connected to every probability that you can fathom. Each probability is a reality occurring simultaneously.

Sometimes we have bleed-through from one of these simultaneous realities. Bleed-through occurs when other probabilities converge, stimulated by the similarity of their originating energy to what is presently occurring. An example of this is past-life recollections. We label them as past-life based on our acceptance of linear time, but the reality is that they are occurring *Now*. Another example is the false memory syndrome, recalling memories of some past incident that might not have truly occurred in this reality. The unconscious mind sometimes believes a suggested incident as a true experience because the emotions attached to it feel real. It does not matter if this incident truly occurred or not, what matters is whether it is real to the individual. In the greater reality of the time continuum, this false memory is a probable reality set in motion, and it has the potential to influence choices in the *Now*.

Not everyone perceives bleed-through or probability through vision or memory, but through other senses such as hearing or feeling. This depends on what internal representation an individual predominately relies upon to experience reality—visual, auditory, kinesthetically, olfactory, gustatory, or a combination of these representational systems. What is important is to realize that it is the acceptance of the possibility that develops the ability.

Collapsing time is the ability to focus on the past or future as *Now*. This creates and facilitates a powerful process for healing emotions. A way to conceptualize this idea of collapsing time is to imagine yourself to be simultaneously an actor and an observer of your life. Seeing yourself as both observer and actor disconnects the emotional hooks with a situation. Call this a state of dissociation. This expanded view of things raises the vibrational frequency and creates a different reality than the reality of being associated with the energy. From this stance, you can feel a similarity with the state of oneness and create a deeper connection to all things. Different oils enhance developing this affinity of being in the past, present, and the future all at once.

Expanding perception to include this reality supports you to make choices that are receptive to Spiritual direction. Accepting that you have an infinite amount of choices for any situation heightens your ability to directly take responsibility for creating and living in a reality based upon your truth.

Vibrational Aromatherapy

Essential oils are the life force of a plant. Like all natural substances they contain spiritual force and energy that affect the spiritual, emotional, mental, physical and etheric bodies, and they affect your vibrations in one way or another. The energy of each individual oil can trigger various states of consciousness, proclaiming to the unconscious mind a willingness to deal with an issue and resolve it. The oils' energies magnetize a vibratory field conducive to feeling supported in love. They provide gentle encouragement to become aware of the thought patterns and emotional patterns that create your reality. Using essential oils strengthens your ability to discern and identify the influences obstructing you from achieving harmony, joy, and balance. They promote a safe environment for you to discover whether your reality is created from your individual truth or if it is being influenced by unconscious re-acting, social consciousness, parents, or peers.

Essential oils help you expand out of the world structured by only five physical senses into one of multi-sensory experiences. A truly multi-sensory human's senses extend beyond physical reality and relies upon intuition as a sense. Intuition is the voice of the Higher Self speaking to the personality. To expand into this perception the mind must have a great ability to accept the nonphysical. Accepting the nonphysical allows the Spirit to become the guiding force in your life. Integrating the Spiritual body with the personality provides the means for spirit to actualize.

Using Essential Oils for Healing

Issues—old traumas, judgments, painful memories—can become stuck in the body, disrupting the energy flow and causing illness. Each discussion of essential oils in the A to Z section includes suggestions for using essential oils with a focused intention and massaging on specific energetic points of the body—your chakras, energy meridians or on hand and foot reflexology points. Using oils on these energy channels enhances the healing process. The following discussions of chakras, meridians and reflexology are a guideline to help point you or your practice partner to the possible location of an energy-blocking issue held in the body. Allow your intuition to guide where and how to use the oils.

Essential oils also help with an intensive meditation technique I call "Embracing Everything into Love." A section in this chapter will describe how to use this technique. "Embracing" is one of the most profound techniques I have used on my spiritual journey. It has greatly helped me to achieve states of Grace and Allowance, bringing peace and restoring balance in my life. Most importantly, it has helped me learn how to love and accept all aspects of myself. By embracing, you initiate and affirm an intention to live in a state of love.

A bath with essential oils is a delightful and powerful method of accelerating healing. An aromatherapy bath can be a quick ten minutes or a two-hour soak, depending on your needs. This chapter includes a discussion of what to expect in a bath and how to prepare a custom bath.

Choosing which essential oil to work with is not always obvious. Intuition is the best tool to use. Anyone can develop their intuitive skills with practice, and we'll also look at a few simple methods of divining the proper essential oils for your healing. Allow your intuition to guide where, how and when to use the oils.

The Chakra System

Chakra is a Sanskrit word that denotes circular movements such as a spinning wheel or vortex. This word is used to describe the dynamic energy centers that connect with Universal spiritual energy, or *prana*, and transform it into physical life force. These energy centers balance, store, and distribute the energies of life and consciousness throughout the body. Each chakra oversees different aspects of life, thoughts, and energy.

The chakras are invisible energetic portals that draw in Universal energy and distribute it via the *nadis*, a network of psychic nerves or channels in the etheric body, into the cells of the physical body. The nadis parallel the autonomic nervous system along the spinal cord of the physical body. Each chakra is a bridge, or energy transformer, that connects the spiritual, etheric (also called the astral) mental, emotional and physical bodies together. The chakras spin at their own specific frequencies. The slowest spinning chakra is the base and the fastest is the crown. (See chart.)

Chakra energy is invisible in the physical realm; it can be monitored, but has no mass or substance of its own. Each individual chakra does, however, have a general location. When the chakras are open, balanced, and cleansed, they offer an opportunity for developing multi-dimensional sensory abilities. The chakras are visible with a developed clairvoyant ability. Yogis in the East (whose language we use) poetically describe the chakras as many-petaled flowers or lotuses. Western Shamans see the chakras as various colored rotating circles or funnels at each particular energy center. The energy of the chakras can be sensed, felt, or seen but it requires shifting to an expanded level of consciousness greater than normal, a state of being that will lead you to discover your true source.

There are many minor energy points in the physical body, and many dormant chakras that will open with an expanded consciousness that allows the physical body to assimilate more light, producing and maintaining a higher frequency of vibration. The thymus chakra, for instance, is opened and developed in individuals expanding their consciousness and awareness. We are mainly concerned with the seven major chakras.

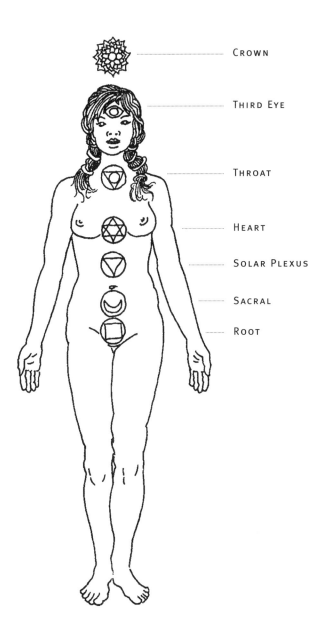

CROWN

THIRD EYE

THROAT

HEART

SOLAR PLEXUS

SACRAL

ROOT

Chakra locations and associations

Each chakra has a location associated with organs or centers of the physical body, a sound, color, and element, as well as aspects of thought, beliefs and consciousness. The base chakra extends down and the crown chakra extends up. The chakras in between have vortexes both to the front of the body and to the back. Most commonly, seven chakras are agreed upon, like the following:

CHAKRA	LOCATION	ORGANS	FUNCTION	ELEMENT	SENSE	SOUND	COLOR
1st Root/ Base	Base of Spine at Perineum	Adrenals Anus Colon	Physical Survival Safety, Birth Grounding	Earth	Smell	"oohm" in tone C	Red
2nd Sexual/ Sacral	Navel Lower Abdomen	Sexual Genitals	Creativity Procreation, Sex	Water	Physical Taste	"ohm" in tone D	Orange
3rd Solar Plexus/ Navel	Bottom Sternum Solar Plexus	Stomach	Power, Will, Self-Empowerment Gut Feelings	Fire, clair-voyance	Sense of Knowing	"ahm" in tone E	Yellow
4th Heart	Above Sternum Over Heart	Heart	Self-Love Acceptance Kindness Compassion	Air	Psychic touch, Empathy	"ah" in tone F	Green/ Pink Rose
5th Throat	Base of Neck (thyroid)	Thyroid	Communication Creativity	Psychic hearing, Clair-audience	Sound	"ehm" in tone G	Blue/ tur-quoise
6th Third Eye/ Brow	Forehead Between and above eyebrows	Pituitary Gland	Higher Self / Goddess-God Inner Vision Intuition Imagination	Light Psychic perception	Sight	"eem" in tone A	Indigo Blue/ Purple

CHAKRA	LOCATION	ORGANS	FUNCTION	ELEMENT	SENSE	SOUND	COLOR
7th Crown	Top of head	Pineal Gland	Spiritual connection to Enlightenment Knowledge Understanding	Astral Projection	Thought	OHM	Violet/White

DORMANT CHAKRA

CHAKRA	LOCATION	ORGANS	FUNCTION	ELEMENT	SENSE	SOUND	COLOR
Thymus	Above Heart over Thymus	Thymus	Divine Love Understanding karmic roles Grace	Ethers	Past/Future Life		Teal

CHAKRAS OUTSIDE OF THE BODY

These become more important with spiritual evolution and the Human DNA structure connects with the Light Body.

8th	Aura			Vibrational Healing		Magnetic Field	

9th	Planet
10th	Solar System
11th	Galaxy
12th	Universe

Each of these relate to the ability to deal with issues on a wider scale. The chakras act as anchor points, forming stable means of interaction with a certain sphere of life.

The Meridian System

While Western medicine separates the body, mind, and emotions, believing them to be independent systems, traditional Chinese medicine treats the whole person, taking into account their emotional, mental, and physical energy states. Traditional Chinese medicine sees the body as a reflection of the order of nature. It is quite similar to the theory of vibrations. *Chi* is the energy force behind all life. Chi is divided into the positive and negative energies of *yin* and *yang*, which are the substances that create all matter. Chi is present in every living organism, and flows through the human body in a system of channels called *meridians*. There are twelve major meridians and each has associations with a specific organ and its functions. In addition to the twelve meridians, there are two major energy vessels, the Governing Vessel and the Conception Vessel.

The flows or blockages of energy in the meridians indicate potential physical, emotional, and mental health problems. Acupuncture is an ancient healing method that uses needles to stimulates energy points on the meridians to release blockages and balance energy. Acupressure stimulates those points with touch. These are both highly effective treatments for physical, mental, and emotional ailments.

To practice these meridian exercises, you will need a partner or client to work on.

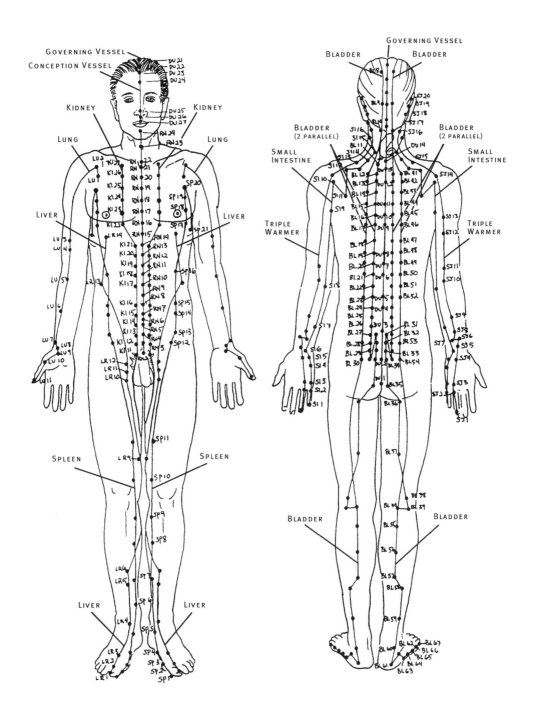

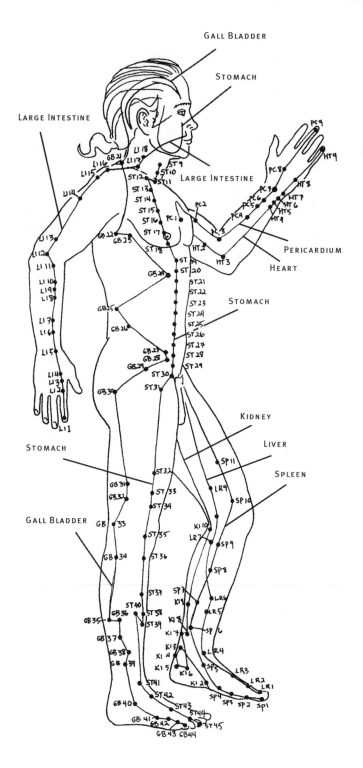

Energizing the meridians

Begin by running your hand lightly over a meridian path from end to end. Refer to the chart of meridians and note whether the natural energy pattern of meridian you are following is Yin or Yang. Yin energy flows up the body from the earth, and Yang energy flows down the body from the sun source.

To clear a meridian of blocked energy, begin by running the energy in the opposite direction of its inherent Yin or Yang energy flow. To energize a meridian, begin by running the energy in the meridian's inherent Yin or Yang direction. This stimulates energy flow and nourishes the organs. You can do all twelve meridians, or just the ones showing signs of being either depleted or over-active. Trace the meridian paths with a steady continuous movement, a couple of times for each meridian.

Do all twelve meridians and the two governing vessels in the following order beginning with the heart:

There is no beginning or end to the cycle of Chi, so we represent the order of the meridians as wheel. As we go around the wheel the flow follows this order on the body. Move along the cycle from the meridian you start to the meridian to the right. If you started with the Lung meridian then move towards the right, which is the Large Intestine and then onto the Stomach. When you reach the Governing Vessel move to Heart and continue.

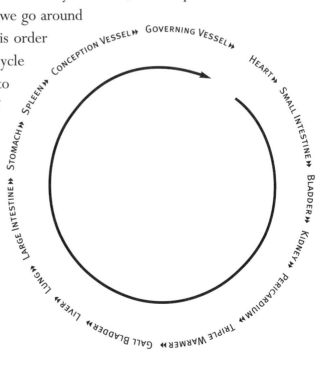

Stimulating meridian points

While giving a massage, you may find the existence of congested energy by feeling for tender points on a meridian. If so, run your hand along the meridian to discover the location of the blocked energy. This is often the most-tender point. To release the block, hold on hand at that site and find another tender point. Locate the second point by moving along the meridian to a point lower on the body. Hold both points for a few seconds, and wait to feel a sensation of heat or a balanced pulse signaling the release. Often one or both of the points will lessen in tenderness. Keep moving up the meridian holding onto two points at a time while visualizing the energy running between them. Hold a stubborn point longer while stimulating other points. Move to the end of the meridian to release obstructions in the energy flow. Then energize the meridian by running the energy with your hand from the bottom of the meridian to the top. Your partner will notice a reduction or disappearance of the tenderness. Often there will be a profound sense of peace and balance.

It is important not to over energize or deplete meridian energy by holding the meridian too long or by energizing the meridian in the wrong direction. To correct this condition, run the energy again by first decreasing the energy. Start at the top of the meridian and flow downwards, then increase energy by reversing the direction.

Attributes of the meridians

The following charts summarize the meridians' attributes and illustrate the energetic relationships influenced by the mental, emotional, physical, and spiritual bodies. Review the charts to become familiar with the energy connections. An understanding of the nature of the meridians' energy and their influences is a very helpful tool for diagnosing physical conditions and emotional issues.

MERIDIAN	HEART (H), (i)	SMALL INTESTINE (Si) (ii)	BLADDER (B) (iii)	KIDNEY (K), (iv)	PERICARDIUM (P), (v)
Yin/Yang	Yin	Yang	Yang	Yin	Yin
Tide	11am-1pm	1-3pm	5-7pm	5-7pm	7-9pm
Chakra	Heart	Sacral	Sacral	Sacral	Heart
Life Aspects	Spirit— Tendency for Growth	Spirit— Discrimination Pure & Impure	Way to Look at Life, Sexuality	To Be in the Moment	Spirit, Feeling Free to Feel Intimacy
Function	Master	Nutritional Assimilation	Liquid Elimination	Water Balance, Metabolism	Protection
Emotion	Joy, Love, Self-confidence, Compassion, Excessive Dreaming, Acceptance	Assimilating Emotions, Desiring, Wanting, Self-Nourishing, Increase Vitality	Receiving, Giving, Supported, Feelings, Relaxed, Accepting	Resolution, Trust, Will Power, Self-assured Embracing Self, Living in the Present, Resting & Storing Energy	Open to Intimate Relationships & Sexuality, Free To Feel, True To Self

Meridian	Heart (H), (i)	Small Intestine (Si) (ii)	Bladder (B) (iii)	Kidney (K), (iv)	Pericardium (P), (v)
Issues	Anxiety Self-Doubt, Sadness, Shock, Hurt, Despair, Nervousness, Emptiness, Abandonment, Over-controlling	Feeling Trapped in Relationships /Life/Body Excessive Talking/ Doing or Inertia	Aggression based on Rage, Fear of Feeling, Terror, Burdened by the World, Overly Tense	Fear, Mistrust, Anxiety, Phobia, Inadequacy, Timid, Panicky Paranoia, Need to be Right, Dominating, Intimidating	Fear To Feel, Persecution, Afraid of Self, Depression
Element	Fire	Fire	Water	Water	Fire
Sense Organ	Tongue/Speech	Tongue/Speech	Ear/Hearing	Ear/Hearing	Tongue/Speech
Body Tissue	Blood Vessels	Blood Vessels	Head Hair, Bones, Marrow	Bone, Marrow, Skeleton	Blood Vessels
Body Fluid	Sweat	Sweat	Urine	Urine	Sweat
Shows Condition	Complexion	Complexion	Head Hair	Head Hair	Complexion
Meridian Disorders	Swollen Glands, Arm painful, weak and numb, Thirst, Insomnia, Stiff Little Finger, Heart disorders, Throat disorders, Irritability, Constipation	Stiff Neck/Arm/ Scapula/ Shoulder, Numb fingers, Hearing loss, Ears ringing, Dim eyesight, Sore throat	Headaches, Tired/ Poor eyes, Clogged sinus, Nosebleeds, Sciatica, Stiff Knee/ Hip/Foot/Toe, Irritability Indigestion, Diarrhea, Hemorrhoids	Tight Chest, Heart Pains, Lung Congestion Asthma, Cough, Leg/Spine Pain Numbness, Hot Feet, Hot/Dry Tongue,	Swollen armpit, Elbow/ Forearm Spasms, Hot Flashes/ Palms Insomnia, Exhaustion, Heart palpitation, Diaphragmatic tightness

Meridian	Triple Warmer (TW), (vi)	Gall Bladder (GB) (vii)	Liver (LV) (viii)	Large Intestine (LI), (x)
Yin/Yang	Yang	Yang	Yin	Yang
Tide	9-11 pm	11 pm-1-am	1-3 am	5-7 am
Chakra	All	Third Eye	Solar Plexus	Root 1
Life Aspects	Spirit moves Emotions to the Heart	Letting Life Flow	Will/Responsibility Ability to Respond to Life	Holding Things In Rather than Letting them Go
Function	Heat Balance	Fat Metabolism, Stores/Secretes Bile	Detoxification, Digestive Absorption, Blood Storage	Elimination of Waste— Diarrhea/ Constipation
Emotion	Warm Family, Feel Emotions, Vitality Ability to Releases Old Roles/ Relationships Courage to Develop New Relationships	Self-Responsibility, Creativity, Flexibility, Accepts Power, Inner-Child Recognized	Re-Birth Self, Integrate Whole-Self, Self-Assertiveness Motivation, Responsible, Will to Do, Expressive, Harmonized, Emotional	Satisfied Feeling, Changes Easily, General Well Being
Issue	Restless/ Anxiety Distracted Depressed, Exhausted, Obsessed, Uncreative, Fixated Attachment	Bitter /Guilt/ Resentful Angry/ Controlling/ Fearful, Blocked Feelings, Incest/Abuse Memories, Takes on Responsibilities, No Will Power	Angry/Frustrated/ Bitter/Vengeful/ Resentful/ Bored/ Depressed, Self-Blame/ Guilty, Stagnated/ Stuck, Self-righteous	Holds Back Feelings, Judgmental, Fear Loss, Depression, Clinging / Possessive, Non-Committal, Grief
Element	Fire	Wood	Wood	Metal
Sense Organ	Tongue/Speech	Eye/Vision	Eye/Vision	Nose/Smell
Body Tissue	Blood, Vascular System	Tendon, Ligaments, Bones, Marrow	Tendon, Ligaments	Skin
Body Fluid	Sweat	Tears	Tears	Mucus
Shows Condition	Complexion	Nails	Nails	Body Hair, Puffy Hands

MERIDIAN	TRIPLE WARMER (TW), (vi)	GALL BLADDER (GB) (vii)	LIVER (LV) (viii)	LARGE INTESTINE (LI), (x)
Meridian Disorders	Swollen cheek, Hearing Loss, Earaches, Shoulder/ Arm/Wrist stiffness and pain, Loss of energy, spontaneous sweating	Eye Problems, Headaches, Bitter taste, Sciatica, Throat/neck/ Joint/Shoulder pain, Poor circulation, Digestive disorders	Puffy/yellow eyes, Diaphragm/ Ribs / Chest tightness, Distorted Vision, Dizzy, Headaches, Migraines, Throat lump, Backache, Abdominal/ Pelvic/Hernias / PMS/vomiting, Frigidity	Stiff Neck, Grind Teeth Facial/ Jaw Tension, TMJ Shoulder/ Arm Pain, Tennis Elbow, Stiff Index Finger/ Hands Block/ Runny Nose, Intestinal disorder Abdominal Pain Diarrhea/Constipate

MERIDIAN	SPLEEN/ PANCREAS (SP), (xii)	LUNG (LU) (ix)	STOMACH (ST) (xi)	GOVERNING VESSEL (GV)	CONCEPTION VESSEL (CV)
Yin/Yang	Yin	Yin	Yang		
Tide	9-11am	3-5am	7-9am	7-9pm	7-9pm
Chakras	Solar Plexus	Throat	Sacral	All	All
Life Aspects	Opinionated, Nourish Self & Not Take the World On	Need to be True to Self	Ability to Embrace all Judgments in Love	Living and Dying	Birth
Function	Blood/Food/ Lymph Digested Transformed Transported	Respiration, Elimination	Digestion— Vomiting/ Belching	Central Nervous System Kundalini	Conception, Circulation/ Sex, Digestion
Emotion	Trust, Empathy, Sympathetic, Loving, Receptive Considerate, Balanced Energy Pleasurable Excitement	Receptive, Open to Flow with Life, Expressive Unattached Self Esteem	Concerned & Connected to Earth, Grounded Nourishing Self	Fully Living Life Contented Loving Life	Acceptance of Power, Conception of Life,

Meridian	Spleen/ Pancreas (SP), (xii)	Lung (LU) (ix)	Stomach (ST) (xi)	Governing Vessel (GV)	Conception Vessel (CV)
Issue	Overly Concern Pity/Worry/ Guilt/Brooding, Mental Fatigue, Lacks Focus, Forgetful, Indifferent Alienated/ Rage Obsessive Judgmental Fears	Rigid, Grief, Anxious, Self-pity, Jealous, Greedy, Selfish, Oppressive Failure, Opinionated	Over Thinking, Worry/Martyr Rebellious Anti-Social Judgmental Unsatisfied Self-centered Low Energy Distracted	Denial, Hysteria, Terror, Nervousness, Impotence, Fear of Death, Addictions	Hysteria, Fears Death, Birth Terror, Addictive Nature
Element	Earth	Metal	Earth	None	None
Sense Organ	Mouth/Taste	Nose/Smell	Mouth/Taste		
Body Tissue	Blood System	Skin, Hair	Muscles, Flesh	Nerves	
Body Fluid	Saliva	Mucus	Saliva		
Shows Condition	Lips	Body Hair	Lips		
Meridian Disorder	Appetite Loss, Nausea, PMS, Abdominal/ Pelvic Pain, Stiff Big Toe, Bunions	Breathing Difficulties, Coughs, Asthma, Congestion Sore Throat, Headaches, Chest Tightness	Digestive Disorders, Red Eyes, Sinus Pain, Toothache, Stiff Neck High Blood Pressure, Knee/Leg/ Shin Pain	Lumbar Pain, Headaches, Fever/Colds/ Allergies, Eye/Nasal Problems Asthma, Nerves Ringing Ears, Stroke, Loss of Consciousness	Throat Obstructions, Hot Flashes, Stomach/ Pelvis/ Genital Swelling & Pain, PMS, Frigidity, Impotence

Attributes of the five elements

The five elements are the cornerstones of traditional Chinese medicine. They are the building blocks of matter. They define the basic laws and principles by which energy manifests. Indispensable life-sustaining relationships originate from each element's specific energy. Each meridian is associated with one of the five elements' qualities.

Element	FIRE	EARTH	METAL	WATER	WOOD
Energetics	Volatile Emotions/ Love	Criticism/ Assurance	Depression/ Enthusiasm	Fear of Living/ Confidence	Frustration/ Patience
Spiritual Manifestation	Spiritual Consciousness	Intelligence	Aura	Aspiration	Soul
Process	Growth/ Acknowledge Spiritual Self	Transformation	Harvest	Storage	Birth
Sound	Laugh	Sing	Weep	Groan	Shout
Emotions	Joy, Hysteria, Sadness	Empathy, Worry, Obsessions Self Absorbed	Grief, Letting Go, Holding On	Discrimination, Paranoia,	Responsible Anger
Personality	Active	Calm	Simple	Constant Movement	Hard Working
Temperament	Emotional Roller Coaster	Obsessed	Anguished	Fearful	Depressed
Injures by Over Use	Using Eyes	Sitting	Lying Down	Standing	Walking
Climate	Hot	Humid/Damp	Dry	Cold	Windy
Season	Summer	Late Summer	Autumn	Winter	Spring
Taste	Bitter	Sweet	Pungent	Salty	Sour
Odor	Scorched	Fragrant	Rotten	Putrid	Rancid
Meridan	SI/H, P, TW	SP, ST	LU, LI	K, B	LV, GB

Hand and Foot Reflexology

Reflexology is a therapy that uses reflex points on the hands and feet to release and rebalance energy. The hands and feet are maps of the entire body and its energy points (see diagrams for location of points of correspondence.) Organs on the right side of the body have their reflex areas on the right side of each hand and foot and organs on the left are located on the left side. Areas of the hands or feet that are tender indicate congestion or imbalance in the corresponding part of the body.

Massaging the oils into the hands and feet can feel very soothing and will stimulate the body's own healing mechanisms. When a part of the body is too sensitive to be touched, the pain can overload the nervous system and create resistance. Reflexology is a gentle approach that relaxes and stimulates healing.

Use the appropriate oil for the energy blockage or specific issue you are working on and massage it into the reflex point. Start with a gentle stroking and slowly increase the pressure to help dissolve the blockage and restore balanced energy circulation. Apply the pressure in a circular pattern if the area is extremely tender. Use both hands to compress areas or use the knuckles to apply a deeper and broader pressure. Listen to the body and let it direct your hands and pressure to the areas needed.

Squeezing and gently pulling and rotating the hand and foot joints helps to stimulate circulation. Unblocking stagnant energy can stimulate the system to pump nourishing blood to all parts of the body and transport toxins from the cells to points of elimination (kidneys, liver, and intestines, for example). Since the feet are furthest from the heart there is a tendency for waste to accumulate there. The stresses of poor fitting shoes and long hours standing can contribute to poor circulation, causing toxins to lodge in the feet and swelling. If this continues for any length of time the toxins begin to calcify and put pressure on the nerve endings. This can become a source of irritation causing more stress in the body. Reflexology helps break up the calcified deposits into smaller pieces that the blood can then transport to points of elimination. This will also relieve pressure on the nerve endings so that tension can be eased and balance and harmony be restored.

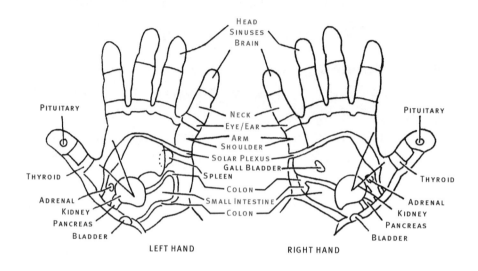

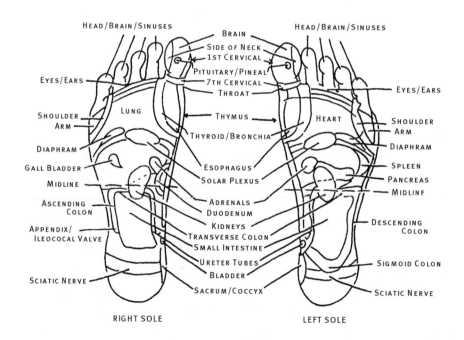

Embracing Everything into Love

There is no right or wrong. Believing so is the grand illusion creating separation from Spirit.

There are no accidents. Every experience has a purpose, and it happens in the right time and place. Life on this plane is about being consciously present in the moment, experiencing and feeling the full spectrum of life. Each of us creates our needed experiences, and each experience serves us in some way. Each experience is an opportunity to move closer to the reality of Spirit. Freewill determines the path we choose.

To reunify Self and Spirit, all experience must be embraced into love without judgment. Embracing creates Divine Allowance; it is a true state of non-judgment. Often the personality's perspective clouds the truth of how a seemingly-negative experience serves a Spiritual purpose. Surrendering all judgment about an issue or experience heals separation, and embracing the situation into love transmutes the energy into wholeness again. The state of Oneness resolves the issues and releases the need to experience it again. Embracing whatever emotions you feel into love validates the experience and aids in healing the separation. Embracing is not the same as forgiveness, which means that something was wrong, and sometimes forgiveness is inappropriate. The difference is that embracing acknowledges your true feelings about a situation, or the reaction stimulated in you which might have roots in some karmic scheme. All emotions are spiritual and you have a right to them but they don't have to keep affecting your life. By embracing them you can discharge and disconnect from the conditioned response giving you choice again. When a charged emotion remains attached to a memory it is a signal that an experience is unresolved.

Working with the energies of essential oils brings to the surface many repressed and denied feelings. Once you are able to get in touch with the painful feelings, using the "Embracing" technique is a profound method of

resolving these issues. Use this technique to transmute any density in your
body or vibrational field. Density is any feeling, action, thought, or response
to a stimulus that is not motivated by love. What is not love is fear, expressed
as feelings of depression, anxiety, anger, hurt, or any emotion that separates
Self from Source.

You can do this exercise anywhere in a relatively short period of time.
When you are learning how to develop this technique, it is very helpful to
write down your beliefs or any uncomfortable feelings or responses that you
feel in the process. It is easier to begin by defining one issue at a time rather
than tackling many at once. Honest introspection leads to discovering the origin of your reaction. Most likely it originates in an unconscious belief created by a judgment, a learned response motivated by fear instead of love, or a
decision created by an experience in a past life, in the womb, or at a tender
age. It could be genealogical. Explore your feelings. They might also surprise
you, especially once you discover how much influence the mass consciousness
has over your perceptions. That realization will allow you to choose to disconnect from that unconscious reality and start shaping a reality of unlimited
possibilities based upon love.

The process requires honest introspection into feelings, actions, responses, and motivations, as well as truthfully acknowledging and taking responsibility for your part in creating the experience. It is also crucial to truthfully
acknowledge all the judgments you have made about yourself and others in
the experience. Admit to yourself exactly how you feel about something and
examine your motives for feeling that way. It is vital to learn not to place
blame on anything or anyone. This allows a greater capacity for acceptance.
The most essential thing is to feel where in the body the beliefs and emotions
the experience has produced.

Charged emotions create energy blocks. These blockages are often felt to
be dense, sticky, and uncomfortable. Charged emotions limit choices because
they stimulate spontaneous reactions that are triggered by familiar energy.
They have a great potential to enact inappropriate responses to present situa-

tions. It is important to search for the origin of these reactions and discover what the purpose or lesson was for this experience. Recognizing how the response has served you and embracing your behavior allows you to chose a reaction that is more appropriate for the situation when the energy occurs again. But sometimes it is not necessary to know the whole story, just that you have those feelings.

It is critical to honestly evaluate the root cause of an issue. Rationalization is a great seduction, hindering our ability to take full responsibility for our part in creating our reality. It prevents us from truly learning our lesson and contributes to repeating the experience. Often the true cause is really only fear perceived by the personality. At first, the truth is hard to admit, but it becomes easier and eventually through practice and experience, you desire the truth because it sets you free.

The Embracing technique

The Embracing technique is the intentional use of breathing, feeling, and visualizing to release energy blocks and transform an experience with love. Give yourself permission to process the energy in any way the body desires. If you are in a group don't pay attention to how others are processing or think that you are being judged or doing it incorrectly.

The breathing process sometimes makes you cough so go ahead and cough up what you need too. If you need to, allow your self to cry or make sounds to express the energy and to help release it. Wailing, moaning, or toning are helpful. If your legs and arms need to move, than do so. Sometimes the energy needs to shake, kick, or punch, to be able to move out. If it is a particularly intense block, a wave of nausea may be felt.

Start by thinking about something that produces an unloving emotional response or is holding your attention, keeping you from being present in the moment. This can be what you want to embrace. It can be a situation, place, or thing; a conflict with someone; a judgment you have about something, someone, or yourself; or a deep secret that causes you discomfort. You might not be able to identify what it is. That's okay. Ask yourself where this energy is stored and feel where it is in your body.

Get into a comfortable position. Inhale the oil that you have chosen and ask that it help you with the issues. Begin focusing on your body. Ask your Higher-self to aide in the process and help you be totally in your body. Center—focus your intention on relaxing each part of your body.

Breathe. Start with slow and deep cleansing breaths. Pull yourself down into your feet. You might begin to feel heavy or feel as if you are sinking into the floor. Align with your Higher-Self and ask to integrate and connect with your emotional, mental, physical, and etheric bodies all at once. This will allow you to better experience the emotions in the physical body. Focus on your intention to Embrace. Feel where that energy is residing in the physical body. Use your breath to help surface the energies and to transmute them through the heart.

Begin to breathe deeply and slowly through your mouth. Pull the energy from the bottom of your feet up into the pit of your stomach. Pull down any heaviness from your head and neck into the stomach. Do long steady breaths while you are feeling the heaviness of the emotion. With slow breaths begin pulling the emotion into a ball.

Define your intention, that you are ready to disconnect from and transmute this energy. Give yourself permission. Return to a slow breath. Visualize where the energy is blocked in your body. Focus on all the reactions or feelings the issue has stimulated in you. Feel in your body all the dense energy connected to the issue. Notice where your body is storing the feelings. Visualize the energy as mud, tar, syrup or maybe strings of energy that are all through your body but attached to the issue. Make a ball by gathering and pulling together all the feelings that are lodged throughout your body attached to the issue. Imagine the feelings as clay and begin rolling it up into the pit of your stomach. Pull all the tendrils from your limbs and head into the ball.

Feel this ball in the pit of your stomach. Notice how heavy and pervasive this energy is and keep focusing the feelings into a ball in the pit of your stomach. Remember to stay out of your head but to feel the experience in your body. It is important to accept how the experience feels instead of rationalizing excuses for your reaction. Remember all reactions serve a purpose.

When the energy feels very dense, start moving it up into your heart, start with a panting breath. Breathe rapidly in and out through your mouth. This rapid breath transmutes the energy. While breathing, ignore sensations of heat, tingling, pain, or dry mouth, just keep breathing and don't fear that you will hyperventilate.

Ask your heart to open up and embrace this energy with love. Begin moving the dense energy that is in the pit up towards the heart. Keep up the rapid panting breath—it will help move the energy into your heart.

Acknowledge and validate whatever it is you are feeling. Grant yourself permission to accept the feeling. Love whatever feelings the experience has produced. Accept that you are human, and you have created the experience to fulfill some lesson.

Open your heart and pull the energy up into it. Embrace it. Imagine the ball as something you cherish. Love it. The heart might be afraid to open for the energy because of the pain it has caused. So visualize your ball of energy as a baby (your inner child) and imagine hugging and loving that baby. Pull the energy up through your heart with love, honoring all the feelings that the experience produced. Acknowledge the experience and the reactions it created.

Keep up the rapid panting breath to help expel the energy through the heart. It may feel stuck or too intense. Keep up the rapid breathing to assist its movement. Ask the heart to embrace this energy with love and remind your heart you are not forgiving what happened, you are just acknowledging that it happened. Tone a sound, any tone will do, to further assist in the transmutation.

Once the energy is embraced you will feeling lightness or laughter will bubble forth and you will definitely feel more at peace. Take responsibility for the learning experience.

If your feel your heart cannot open enough to embrace the issue then visualize dropping the ball of dense energy and watch it shatter into hundreds of pink bubbles of joy. These bubbles will expand, filling your being with love.

If you can not allow yourself to feel then just acknowledge the existence of the density.

Breathe deeply while you visualize loving yourself. With enough practice focusing your intent, you will begin feeling safe enough to learn how to feel again and be secure in allowing feelings. *Denying feeling only creates pain.* The experience of pain is the physical body communicating that it is not feeling loved. Feeling is truly much easier and joyful.

If you need to know what the lesson of the experience was, just ask for clarity. If it is necessary to consciously acknowledge the lesson, do so. If it is not necessary to know consciously, just accept that you have learned the lesson and it is complete. Once the lesson is complete, it becomes unnecessary to experience it again unless you choose to do so. Now you can choose a reaction that is more appropriate to the current situation, a choice generated in the Now, and not out of the past.

The next step is to visualize yourself as a child and truly love that child. Connect your heart chakra to the heart chakra of your Inner Child. Embrace that child into your heart without judgment. You will begin to feel that density move up into the Heart chakra so that it can be transmuted into love.

You will know that the density has transmuted because the old belief is not necessary any longer. Your perspective changes about the issue. Many times there is a group of beliefs that will flood your consciousness. Just ask to feel the emotion and love each experience you had.

The greatest service of the Embracing Everything into Love technique is it teaches you the allowance and acceptance to fully love and honor Self without judgment. Learning to love Self actualizes Spirit to manifest on the Earth Plane. It aligns you with your Divine purpose and fulfills your mission to live life in a loving manner.

The Aromatherapy Bath

Essential oil baths are a powerful transformational tool for healing and raising vibration. Aromatherapy baths are phenomenally successful in treating numerous conditions such as asthma, allergies, insomnia, sore muscles, arthritis, and hyperactivity. An aromatherapy bath can detoxify the body of environmental pollutants as well as drug and alcohol toxins. The baths also successfully treat the emotional and mental bodies, releasing issues such as depression, anger, grief, fear, anxiety, fatigue, and numerous other emotions. The spiritual body aligns with the physical through the baths, enhancing the ability to receive guidance from Source.

Instead of a full soaking bath, sometimes a simple hand or foot bath can address conditions such as rheumatism, arthritis, dermatitis, psoriasis, and dry and flaky skin. A spinal soak is a short—only eight to ten minutes are required—but very powerful bath that clears psychic dirt from the aura and balances all the major meridians. Prepare a spinal bath by adding two cups of apple cider vinegar into four inches of very hot water, then lie in the bath soaking the spine and neck. You may add essential oils to the vinegar.

A plaster of red clay or mustard taken before an essential oil bath can greatly enhance the healing effects. The action of red clay helps poisons and toxins release from the physical body. Red clay is feels very grounding. To prepare a plaster, mix the clay with water to form a pasty consistency, then lather on the body. To increase its effects, lie out in the sun till it dries, then wash off the clay. Follow with an essential oil bath.

A mustard plaster is warming to the body and helps release mucus from the lungs. Use this plaster when congestion is present. Prepare the herb in same manner as red clay. Lather the paste on the chest and back, let it dry, wash it off, and follow with a bath.

Preparing an essential oil bath

Begin by creating a soothing and nurturing environment by using dim lights, candles, flowers and soft music. Allow enough time for the bath as well as time to relax afterwards. This extra time completes the energetic changes and aids in stabilizing the new energy.

Use an intuitive technique to determine the length of your bath, which can last from 15 minutes to two hours. Make the water as hot as is tolerable. Begin by adding a base ingredient to the bath water. Base ingredients work synergistically with the essential oils to accelerate healing effects. Most ingredients can be purchased in bulk at a health food store. Dowse or pendulum for specific ingredients and quantity, the usual quantity ranges from one-half to three cups. Base ingredients are:

SEA SALT—clears the subtle bodies or auric field, releases anger and balances energy.

RAW APPLE CIDER VINEGAR—clears emotional toxins from the subtle bodies; is nurturing to the body, hair and skin.

BAKING SODA—releases toxins from the physical body. It also removes cobalt, plutonium and radioactive isotopes from the body.

CHLORINE BLEACH—detoxifies the lymphatic system by removing petrochemicals, drug deposits, heavy metals and radioactive isotopes. After being x-rayed, take a chlorine soak followed by a combined sea salt and baking soda bath.

FRESH LIME JUICE—balances the subtle bodies, healing any rips and holes in the aura.

CHAPARRAL TEA—a general cleanser, and an essential bath for those living in a city with air pollution. It detoxifies the blood, kidneys, liver, lymph and thymus. To make the tea, boil one-quarter cup of dried herb in a quart of water for approximately ten to fifteen minutes and strain it before adding to the bath.

GINGERROOT—clears toxins from the lungs, and from the body by its ability to promote sweating. Cut up the fresh root and prepare a tea as above.

RED CLOVER—assimilates and purifies the subtle body field and pulls toxins from the physical body. Prepare a tea as above.

Add your essential oil or oils to the water. Be certain to check the precautions for each oil and be aware of possible side effects. Some of the oils are inappropriate for children or during pregnancy. Stir the oils well in the tub. Get in, submerging the total body. If the tub is too small, alternate between sitting up and raising the feet out of the tub.

Add additional ingredients, if desired. These may be flower and mineral essences, Bach remedies, crystals or other special objects. Have a cold-press oil such as almond, olive, or safflower on hand to rub on the skin to alleviate any burning sensations. Be sure to mix ingredients before totally immersing yourself in the water. If possible do not shower off the oils after the bath. This will ensure the effects continue processing. It is important to focus on a clear and defined purpose for the bath. While bathing, do a meditation or visualization technique to enhance healing.

You can use some of the Embracing Everything into Love techniques during the bath. Always ask Spirit to be present and invite the healing Angels to participate in your life. Surrendering to Spirit accelerates healing of issues and promotes Spiritual growth. Often repressed emotions and memories will surface during the bath. To increase results, ask for insights into lessons challenging your life. Take responsibility for creating the life experiences and grant permission for accepting the issue in love to resolve its need to be maintained. Focus your intent, feel the dense energy, and embrace the issue by validating the feelings attached to it. Then bring the energy up into your heart. Embrace the density and feel it transform in your heart.

Granting the body permission to release suppressed memories allows for past experience lodged in the cellular memory to begin being recalled and healed. This trauma might manifest in the form of whelps, burns, rashes, or be felt as burning sensations. Do not be alarmed. If your body becomes trapped in the past, you need to state the present date, remind your body that was the past, and it now resides in the present time. If burning occurs later in the bath, this is a sign that density is being transmuted. Ask your body to release in a gentler fashion and call upon Divine Grace to assist the process. If this does not work, rub a cold press oil on the area or add it to the bath to overcome intense burning. If intense burning occurs in the beginning of the bath, this is a sign of resistance to change or denial. Try initiating a dialogue for developing a friendship with the body and the inner-child to create greater self-trust.

Many people experience spontaneous crying, screaming, laughing, or other emotional outbursts, while others may have visions or memories of past and present trauma or other revealing information that will assist in transforming behavioral patterns and attitudes. Sometimes the room fills with the Devic energies of the oils, a true blessing. Focus on the future you want to create or the abilities you want to initiate and heighten. All is possible by asking and being open to receive. Ask to release anything obstructing the ability to receive what you want.

Be prepared to work through the issues. The processing does not end by getting out of the bath. Sometimes it goes on for days. Some baths will surface issues, while others soothe and resolve issues. Sometimes a series of baths are called for. You will need to intuit how many baths to take, how many days apart they need be, whether they are all made with the same ingredients, and the length of time for each bath.

Choosing Essential Oil Combinations Intuitively

If you are seeking to heal physical symptoms, choosing an oil will likely be easy. However, if you are looking for information about unconscious and possibly repressed sources of physical, emotional, or mental difficulties, you will need to use your intuition.

Intuition is the skill receiving knowledge directly from Source, without evident rational thought or inference. Intuition bypasses the distorting filter between the unconscious and the conscious minds. It is the language of communication with the unconscious, physical, emotional, and spiritual bodies. Intuition is a skill, which means it can be developed and mastered with practice.

Begin by simply asking what oil you will need. Any person with adequate trust in their intuition can easily choose the oils needed just by noticing the oils that attract their attention and trusting that information. Intuitive flashes can be perceived through any and all five senses, as hot and cold feelings, or by noting changes and differences of sensations such as energy pulsing in vibrational frequencies. Pay close attention and distinguish the subtle differences.

Use the list provided in the A to Z of oils. When reading the names, do any jump out at you? Experiment by running your finger down the list. Does it stop at a candidate? You will possibly feel hot, cold, or feel the tingling of your hair "standing on end." The body will feel some type of vibrational sensation.

Talk to your unconscious mind and ask it to emit a consistent symbol, particular color, particular sensation, or sound that identifies a yes and no. You can consciously develop this language by defining symbolic representation and affirming its meaning. You need to practice consistently, so the symbol becomes an established pattern that will easily enact unconsciously.

Begin by using the sense that you think is easiest for you to access, visualizing or hearing, for example. Try closing your eyes and slowly moving your finger down the list. Your mind's eye may see "yes" or "no" spelled out. Choose specific colors to represent which is a yes and which a no, and tell this to your unconscious mind. When you see a color with your inner-eye, this indicates a possible choice. You may tell your unconscious to listen for information: hearing a yes or no, a buzzing, thumping, or some other distinctive noise. Once a sense is mastered, try heightening another sense.

Another easy method is to ask the unconscious mind to address an issue by opening a book to a meaningful page and reading it. You will often find information relevant to your issues. Then close your eyes and flip through the pages, stopping at the one that feels right.

If you have narrowed the oils down to several choices, you may use the very easy pendulum method to decide. A pendulum can be made of anything—a paper clip and string, or a chain with a pendant at the end. Hold the end of the chain so the weight can swing freely. The direction the pendulum swings in answers the yes/no question. To establish which direction is yes and which is no, ask a yes or no question that you already know the answer to. Then notice the direction the pendulum swings. Usually it will be in an up-or-down motion for one answer, and side-to-side for the other.

If the pendulum swings in a circular direction, it might mean maybe, or that the question is not clearly phrased for a yes or no answer. It could indicate that you are not certain what your question actually is. It is possible to get a false reading by concentrating on an outcome. Clearly focus your mind on the question, not on what you desire the outcome to be. Practice this method till you feel confident in its effectiveness

If you have some oils on hand already you may use your body as the pendulum by holding bottle of oil and asking if it is the correct oil to use at this time. If you think you have identified the correct oil but do not have it available, write the name on a piece of paper and hold it on your heart chakra.

Stand up, feet apart, and clear your mind. Ask a question that can be answered with a yes or no response. Notice the direction that your body naturally falls toward: "yes" is forward and "no" is backward. This is a wonderful technique to use for choosing all sorts of things, and can be done without calling much attention to you, especially when in a public situation. Experiment and note whether there is a difference when asking questions with your eyes open or closed. It can be highly effective to close your eyes when seeking deeply repressed information stored in the unconscious. The open eyes help access information that the conscious mind has influence over.

Pendulums can be used with radiant charts that provide more information than simply yes or no. Hold a pendulum still in the center, then ask the question. It will answer by continuously swinging over the correct option.

The Essential Oils A to Z

A Note of Precaution

Aromatherapy requires you to take responsibility for your healing process and treatment. Exercise a little caution and the benefits can be tremendous.

Essential oils are so highly concentrated that a little goes a long way. Compared to the toxins we ingest and the environmental pollution we live in, aromatherapy is relatively safe. But undesirable side effects can result from ignorance and overdosing.

When using essential oils, you must consider the oil's purity. Since it takes an immense quantity of raw material to yield a small amount of pure essential oil, pure plant oils are often diluted with synthetic base oils or otherwise reconstituted with less pure and less expensive synthesized oils that contain the same chemical constituents. Turpentine is frequently used to dilute oils, which may falsely reclassify irritating oils as non-irritants. Be sure to obtain your oils from a reputable source and buy the highest quality possible. Unfortunately, the price of the oil will often be an indicator of its quality. If you must buy less expensive oils do not use more to obtain the desired results and especially don't use them internally.

Inhaling oils is relatively non-toxic. Most discomfort comes from not diluting the oil before applying it to skin. Essential oils are best diluted in another pure cold pressed plant oil such as almond, olive, or safflower. Always dilute oils first, and check for an allergic reaction before extensive use. To find allergies, rub the diluted oil on the inner wrist and wait 15 minutes, then check for a reaction. Recommended dilutions and other precautions are noted in the discussion of each oil. Some oils photosensitize the skin and can cause dermatitis. You must keep exposure to sunlight at a minimum when using these oils as they can create redness, lesions, or a sunburn.

Be extra cautious when using essential oils on children and always dilute essential oil for children more than you would dilute for use on an adult. Do not use any potentially irritating oil on children and be especially careful of their sensitive skin. Always use the purest oil available.

The greatest potential hazard is ingesting oils. While internal use of essential oils for treating illness is a common practice in countries such as France, Germany, England, Italy, India, and China, I do not advocate taking the oils internally to achieve the results described in this book. If you choose to use oils internally, ingest essential oils under the supervision of a qualified aromatherapist or physician who has access to medicinal grade oils. You must use only those oils labeled medicinal grade internally. For oils to be effective internally, the treatment must follow a regimented synergistic formula. Unsupervised internal use of the oils can be more harmful than beneficial. Never give young children or babies essential oils internally.

List of Oils

Allspice	Lime
Basil	Marjoram
Bergamot	Myrrh Gum
Black Pepper	Myrtle
Cajeput	Neroli
Calamus Root	Nutmeg
Camphor of Borneo	Orange (Sweet)
Cardamon Seed	Palmarosa
Carrot Seed	Patchouli
Cedar Leaf (Cedarwood, Thuja)	Pennyroyal
Celery Seed	Peppermint
Chamomile	Petitgrain
Cinnamon	Pine
Citronella	Rose
Clary Sage	Rosemary
Clove Bud	Rosewood
Cypress	Rue
Eucalyptus	Sage (Wild Sage or
Fennel	Dalmatian Sage)
Fir, Siberian	Sandalwood
Frankincense	Sassafras
Geranium (Rose)	Savory
Ginger	Spearmint
Grapefruit	Tangerine (Mandarin)
Helichrysum	Tarragon
(Everlasting, Immortelle)	Tea Tree
Hyssop	Vanilla
Juniper	Vetiver
Laurel Leaf (Bay Laurel)	Wintergreen
Lavender	Wisteria
Lemon	Ylang-Ylang
Lemon Grass	

ALLSPICE   *Pimenta dioica – Myrtaceae*
Transformations

Key: Speaking your truth. Allspice can help you gain the ability to express what is true to your heart. Courage for creative self-expression leads to more comfortable interaction with others. Detachment from the emotional charges of unpleasant childhood or past-life memories stimulates emotional healing and generates more self-love.

Growth and healing issues

The essence of Allspice assists problems of poor self-esteem, low self-confidence, and frustration and anger, which block self-expression. These issues are often rooted in feelings of feeling unloved, abandonment, and the self-rejection that often occurs from keeping toxic family secrets that generate shame and emotional detachment. When the environment is not a supportive and safe place for self-expression, then procrastination, introversion, and shy behaviors are a usual result.

Energetic influences on the bodies and chakras

Allspice releases the energy blockages and distortions created by unfulfilled childhood needs and held in the root and sacral chakras. Releasing these energy distortions allows the throat chakra to open and truth to be spoken.

Energetics of the oil

The energy of Allspice feels similar to the startling sensation of being sprayed with cold water on a hot afternoon. Allspice oil's energy rejuvenates and stimulates the desire for action on the physical plane. It awakens the desire to search for and embody your Soul's true essence.

Energetically, Allspice surfaces feelings of rejection and anger lodged in the etheric pancreas. Repeated feelings of failure may discourage you so much that they feel it is hopeless to attempt anything. These emotions are easily repressed in your emotional body. Allspice can surface memories of being persecuted or burned for speaking your truth. Allspice oil can help motivate those caught up in procrastination. It also empowers a shy person to begin feeling more at ease with social interaction. Introverts could use Allspice to help them generate the courage to feel comfortable in social gatherings. Allspice releases repressed grief usually held in the physical lungs and in the emotional body, allowing cleansing tears to flow. On an energetic level, working with intent and the warming energy of this oil helps to gently transmute unconscious memories.

Allspice releases energy distortions created by feeling and believing that your childhood emotional needs were never fulfilled. Growing up in a family where your emotional needs were unfulfilled can generate poor self-esteem and hinder the ability to love yourself and develop self-confidence. This energy distortion is held in the root and sacral chakras, which can then suppress the throat chakra and stifle your ability to express your emotions. Stammering, stuttering, or other speech impediments may even manifest, compounding the problem, ultimately stifling any ability to ask that your needs to be met. The intense frustration felt in blocked chakras can manifest as a lack of self-confidence, in aggression, or in defensive behaviors.

Toxic family secrets hinder a person's ability to express themselves. Keeping secrets early in life starts a pattern of hiding feelings, which generates shame. A person carrying the burden of secrets finds it difficult to relate truthfully to the world, which eventually stops the person from talking about feelings. This gives the unconscious further permission to suppress unpleasant childhood experiences. Using Allspice in meditation allows you to acknowledge painful experiences. Taking an honest look at the situations that have influenced your life is a step towards healing. Once suppressed energy is acknowledged and embraced, you may create new patterns. The energy distortions in the first and second chakras begin healing, stimulating the release of energy obstructions in the throat chakra. This clearing helps you to begin speaking your truth from the heart, and encourages the discovery of new mediums of expression. Allspice helps to unleash the creative energy of expression, allowing it to manifest in a variety of ways.

Using the oil for transformation

Using Allspice oil on the stomach meridian releases obstructions in the energy that help overcome anti-social behavior. Additionally, the Allspice energetically expands the lung meridian, which anchors greater self-esteem and permits a freer expression of self. To open throat chakra energy, gently stroke and massage Allspice into the neck. Inhaling the oil while toning, sounding mantras, or chanting helps the throat energy. Greater release comes when massaging Allspice into the lung meridian while stimulating the lung reflex points on the hands and feet. Massage the oil into the back of the legs to stimulate the bladder meridian to release suppressed emotions.

Hold the occiput (located at the base of the skull where the neck connects) to acknowledge feelings of grief or other repressed or unconscious memories. Cradling the back of the head in one hand while the other hand touches the third eye point energetically releases energy blocked by denied emotions. Allow intuition to determine how long you should hold the points for achieving balance and well being.

Using the throat reflex points found under the big toe on either foot helps to stimulate self-expression energy. Apply oil to these throat points and hold with deep pressure. There are also throat reflex points located on the hands at the base of either thumb. Stimulate these points in the same manner. Massaging along the conception vessel also helps to clear any obstructions in the throat chakra.

Precautions

Allspice can irritate the skin and mucous membranes and is photosensitizing; keep exposure to sunlight at a minimum. Dilute 1-10 drops in 2 ounces of carrier oil. Use only 1-5 drops in a bath. Do not use this oil on children or infants. Be cautious of the purity of Allspice oil because it is often diluted with synthetics or less expensive constituents.

AMYRIS   *Amyris Balsamifera-Rutaceae*
Transformations

Key: Awareness of one's natural cycles and rhythms. Amyris helps you develop an understanding of what it means and feels to be in "Divine Right Timing." Amyris anchors the state of openness that promotes new thoughts and allows new ideas to form and encourages the realization that you have the power to create and direct your life and destiny. Amyris saturates the aura with creativity, which in turn attracts abundance. Unconscious spiritual truths are more easily realized. The faith that goodness is prevalent in life is restored. Amyris aids in building a foundation of trust between the unconscious and conscious mind.

Growth and healing issues

Amyris helps you recognize the preconceived judgments held and validated by the collective consciousness. This oil energetically aids in releasing stereotypical prejudices by helping you realize that it is not wrong or bad for others to have different perceptions or customs. This reduces the discomfort of being out of rhythm with others. Amyris encourages exploration into other dimensions and new realms of thought. It subdues the logical mind and its resistance to accepting, allowing, or validating intuitive impressions and provides support in fulfilling your spiritual destiny.

Energetic influences on the bodies and chakras

Amyris stimulates vibrant physical health by releasing physical and etheric toxins that distort your energy. It regenerates the skin and slows the aging process. Amyris works with the dreaming body to process and acknowledge spiritual truths. It stimulates kundalini energy to move up and out through the heart chakra. Amyris helps you laugh at yourself.

Energetics of the Oil

The word Amyris suggests "amour" or love. Amyris helps you to love yourself. Amyris helps you perceive the magic working in your life and acknowledge unconscious spiritual truths. It restores an innocent outlook on life and generates a renewed sense of faith. Amyris helps you recognize unconscious emotions and encourages you to establish new responses. The knowledge that you have the power to change the course of your life frees you and makes life a more joyous experience.

Amyris soothes and nourishes the heart. It calms rebellious passions by releasing inappropriate attachments, which in turn releases the fears that create states of limitation. The calming energy anchors you in a state of openness, allowing new thoughts and ideas to form. This releasing and calming helps you overcome self-absorption and self-centeredness.

Amyris is a useful oil for dreamers, philosophers, musicians, and artists who draw upon creative Source energy. Use this oil to stimulate astral travel and dream work. Amyris oil synergistically enhances the moon's energy to stimulate the unconscious mind, heightening intuition, psychic talents, creativity, and imagination. The alignment with moon energy stimulates your awareness of the ebbs and tides of energy, leading to a greater understanding of your life cycles and biorhythms. Increasing your awareness of patterns or cycles—such as time to learn, time to absorb and assimilate, time to rest or act, time to teach or create—helps you make more fluid transitions through these cyclic stages. Being attuned to your rhythms keeps you present in the moment, and delivers you into the state of Divine Right Timing.

Energetically, the oil stimulates the movement of the kundalini energy coiled at the base of your spine up into the heart chakra. This flow of energy promotes a feeling of heart-centered sensuality, allowing you to experience sexuality with more conscious awareness. Amyris saturates the aura with fertility, which attracts abundance and creativity.

The Amyris plant is native to Haiti and other Caribbean islands and Central America. The oil embodies the energy of the discovery of the New World and the exploration into new dimensions and thought. It helps you gain access to memories of the Renaissance, a period of birthing new thought. It works with the energies of the planet Venus to inspire love, and encourages seeing the beauty in all things.

Using the oil for transformation

Amyris energy stimulates physical healing by releasing physical and etheric toxins. It clears the intestinal flora of toxins. The oil regenerates the skin and is especially effective on wrinkles and aging. Amyris energy slows the aging process by addressing the issues and beliefs that promote aging. Slowing down and being in the moment contributes to a more relaxed demeanor. Learning to be gentle and more compassionate with yourself frees your spirit and lessens the burden of aging.

The energy of Amyris is very loving and generates self-acceptance, bringing the energy of grace into your life. This loving grace stimulates the ability to laugh at yourself. Use the oil on the heart meridian to feel more at peace with life. Massage into the spine and up into the base of the neck to unlock the kundalini and unleash creativity. Rub onto the stomach and large intestine meridians to release pent-up sexual frustrations. It will help you feel more grounded let you delight at being in the present.

Precautions

Amyris is fairly safe; check for allergy before using. Use 15-30 drops in 2 ounces of a base oil.

ANGELICA ROOT   *Angelica archangelical – Umbelleferae*
Transformations

Key: Awakens multi-dimensional sensory awareness. Angelica helps you embrace Divine Grace. It stimulates compassionate understanding of the state of separation from Spirit. Angelica helps you acknowledge your responsibility for creating the challenging situations in your life and recognize the purpose these experiences serve, which ultimately bridges the separation from Spirit. Greater integration with Spirit increases self-acceptance and self-actualization. Changing your perception allows you to assimilate new energy frequencies. Feeling secure in yourself stimulates a greater acceptance of the diversity of life.

Growth and healing issues

Angelica helps you recognize the emotional and relationship patterns that hinder your growth. It breaks through the denial that closes your heart to deeply rewarding emotional connections with others. You begin to perceive Angelic presences. Angelica initiates multi-dimensional awareness and awakens a magnitude of possibilities, helping you to realize your spiritual purpose. Angelica teaches the lesson that all time is now. This fundamental lesson collapses time and heals the charged emotions that disrupt harmony in your relationships with yourself, your environment, and others.

Energetic influences on the bodies and chakras

Angelica expands the heart chakra. It aligns the third eye with the physical eyes to allow new perceptions. Aligning inner and outer sight encourages greater creativity and self-expression. Opening the thymus chakra stimulates recollection of past life experiences and recognition of how these experiences influence your present life. Embracing past-life experiences releases their influence over your judgment and increases your ability to love yourself and acknowledge that you are living in the perfection of Spirit.

Energetics of the oil

The name Angelica oil invokes images of Angelic Beings. Angelica encourages your Spirit to freely soar in its true, unencumbered state of bliss. Angelica breaks the constriction of limiting thoughts such as fantasy images of love created by social conditioning and movie images. Angelica oil awakens your ability to feel emotions more truly, allowing heart chakra energy to expand. It also heightens clairvoyance.

Angelica energy increases awareness of Angelic presences. Developing a sense of our Angelic essence allows us to feel the energy connecting all things in a state of oneness, enhancing our ability to perceive the Angelic Realm and own it as a part of our reality. The simple knowing of Angels allows their energy to enrich our lives in many ways. Their presence induces feelings of security, enabling a state of Divine surrender—integration with Spirit without the loss of individuality.

Angelica stimulates the right brain, inspiring creativity, intuition, and the development of artistic talents. Angelica oil promotes seeing from a different perspective, broadens narrow points of view, and lets us perceive the beauty in everything through the physical eye. Aligning the physical and inner eyes creates an awareness of magnitude of beauty in and around our lives. Angelica allows us to appreciate how truly wondrous life is.

Use of Angelica with the intention of becoming more focused expands the heart's capacity to feel and heightens compassion toward yourself and others. Developing compassion increases your comprehension of humanity's pain at being separated from Spirit.

Angelica oil's energy stimulates the thymus chakra located above the heart chakra behind the breastbone. The thymus controls the immune system. Many immune disorders or diseases come from judgment of the Soul's journey. Learning to take responsibility for all your actions develops and opens the thymus chakra. Being able to comprehend the roles we play for each other in the game of life develops the thymus chakra. This important chakra, recently discovered, influences the assimilation of new energy frequencies and the ability to be multidimensional.

Angelica oil motivates the search for new attitudes about relationships, opening new avenues of expressing and relating, allowing relationships to grow and transform. This includes our relationships with others, our relationship with ourselves, and even with life itself. Angelica also inspires understanding the relationships with our male and female selves. Most importantly, it enhances our understanding of our relationship to the multitude of probabilities.

Using the oil for transformation

Use Angelica on the pituitary point on the big toe and on the thymus point of the feet to expand perception. Oil massaged on the brow opens and expands the third eye energy. Rubbing the oil on the front and back of the heart chakra will begin to soften the heart's rigid feelings. Using the oil on the heart meridian helps to establish the joy of being. Angelica oil on the triple warmer meridian generates more energy into the heart which releases shoulder stiffness. The key physical body points pertaining to relationship issues are the back of the shoulders behind the heart next to the shoulder blades. (A good guideline to remember is the right side of the body pertains to male issues, and the left side to female issues.) People who carry stress in their upper backs experience relief by using the oil on the Angelic "wing bone" area on either shoulder blade joint where the Angelic body anchors into the physical body.

Precautions

Avoid using Angelica during pregnancy. Diabetics should be cautious of this oil. Angelica is generally non-irritating; to be certain, check for a reaction. Use 15-30 drops in 2 ounces of a base oil. Angelica is photosensitizing, keep exposure to sunlight to a minimum.

STAR ANISE   *Illicium verum — illiciaceae*
Transformations

Key: Understanding cosmic knowledge. Star Anise awakens you to unconscious encoding, transforming old thought patterns into new paradigms and heightening your intuition. Shifts in your perception allow greater reception of intuition and guidance from the Source and the Unseen Realms. You acquire the ability to interpret encoded cosmic knowledge held in the five-pointed star and other sacred geometric forms. A more grounded experience of cosmic knowledge eases into your present physical reality, stimulating your personality to integrate with Spiritual direction.

Growth and healing issues

Star Anise activates dormant encoding that opens new paradigms of cosmic thought and manifests greater conscious awareness. It amplifies and heightens clairaudience, clairvoyance, telepathic, and intuitive abilities. Star Anise helps you recognize resistance to change and the constrictions in your energy caused by fears such as doubt, anxiety, frustration, and insecurity. Freeing this energy is instrumental to shifting your reality and becoming motivated by spirit.

Energetic influences on the bodies and chakras

Star Anise releases constrictions in the etheric body caused by fear, enabling the physical body to feel more secure and harmonious with life. It aligns the chakras with the new frequencies to consciously ground this energy and manifest it into your physical reality. The crown chakra expands, lessening any resistance to or discomfort with these new, lighter frequencies of energy. The new frequencies describe what is known as the light body, which has a faster and higher octave of frequency than the dense frequency of fear. Opening and aligning the chakras with the light body raises the physical body's vibration, which can then harmoniously assimilate the increased energy flow.

Energetics of the oil

Anise stimulates the feeling of reverence, the feeling of standing on sacred ground or a power spot. The energetics of Anise open remembrance of cosmic knowledge. The star-shaped Anise seed symbolically embodies the star-seeds of cosmic knowledge in the unconscious mind, awaiting germination. Anise oil's energy heightens your intuition to let you receive guidance from Source and not be overwhelmed by it. The universal knowledge and energy you receive through Anise is grounded and ready for practical application in sensing and developing innate telepathic skills.

Anise stimulates the development of clairaudience, the ability to hear your inner sources and the Soul's harmonics. Anise creates a sense of security by freeing constrictions in the etheric body generated by fear energies—doubt, anxiety, frustration, etc. Unrestricted, harmonious energy flows into the physical body. This energy, called prana, is transformed into physical energy.

Anise awakens the sacred encodings of the five-pointed star form, knowledge instrumental to stepping out of third-dimensional density. We recognize how critical it is to understand the reasons for an experience, and the impact those lessons have on creating possible choices. Experiences are created to teach lessons for spiritual growth. Learning a lesson completes the need to recycle old patterns and generates movement towards more harmonious experiences directed by Spirit.

Anise awakens knowledge encoded in other forms of sacred geometry. Life is patterned from the signature of these forms. Having an awareness of form heightens psychic perception and stimulates inherent telepathy and knowing. Encoded geometric forms stimulate discovery of unconscious thought patterns and influence the shift of old realities into new paradigms. When you remember how to consciously love, these encodements make miracles common occurrences.

When these new energies are stimulated, their intensity can feel like sharp pains in the head, possibly creating a headache. Resistance to change intensifies the pain. Strong resistance can create blockage or misalignment of the chakras, creating confusion in the physical body. Anise oil helps realign the chakras to receive the new frequencies of energy. Realignment diminishes fears of shifting consciousness and is instrumental to developing psychic skills like telepathy and hands on healing. Anise also balances the etheric energies coming into the physical body, prompting cosmic thoughts to manifest into your present physical reality.

Using the oil for transformation

Anise oil placed on the crown chakra and behind the ears tunes the etheric ear to new frequencies. Massaging the oil in the kidney meridian also opens the inner ear. Use the oil on the temple to ease body tension created by energetic transmissions from Source. Massaging Anise oil into the governing, triple warmer, and conception meridians helps align the seven major chakras. Inhaling the oil is soothing to the bronchial tubes. Assimilating each breath into the physical body opens the power center of the throat while expanding the heart. Anise also stimulates digestion, and grounds Spirit into the physical body. Cleansing the solar plexus chakra with Anise will clarify intuition. Use the oil on the gallbladder and liver meridians to help adjust to the energies. Stimulate the pituitary and hypo-thymus reflexology points in hand and foot to help the crown and third eye open. Use on the thymus chakra, located above the heart in the middle of the chest, to more easily assimilate memories of other life times and parallel dimensions. Rubbing Anise into the soles of the feet will help to anchor the information by grounding through the foot chakras while expanding your perception.

Precautions

Do not use this oil on children or infants. Be cautious of this oil's purity because it is often diluted with synthetics or less expensive constituents. Anise oil is fairly non-irritating; use 15-30 drops in 2 ounces of a base oil but check for an allergic reaction before extensive use.

BASIL   *Ocimum spp – Labiatae*

Transformations

Key: Actualizing Spirit. Basil encourages us to accept responsibility for our intentions and to realize what reality we are creating. Living life with responsibility and integrity promotes making more conscious choices which ultimately gives us the power to manifest the reality we desire. This opens pathways for more spiritual energy to actualize into the physical. Personality becomes a vehicle for expressing spirit. Basil's vibrational frequencies increase the multi-dimensional consciousness that awakens our ability to hear the call to service, opening the way to live more in the moment and able to honor all forms of life.

Growth and healing issues

Basil raises issues of low self-esteem, self-limitation, low self-worth, and the need to judge and be in control regardless of the consequences. Learning to discern and accept true spiritual guidance diminishes doubt, worry, depression, and other fears. Basil generates enthusiasm for life by releasing the need to carry the unnecessary and limiting burdens of anxieties.

Energetic influences on the bodies and chakras

Basil activates dormant encoding in the brain and opens new pathways for energy to assimilate. The physical body is able to better interface with the light body energy and consciousness. This realignment helps us realize how much our emotional baggage limits us. The physical body begins to actualize more ethereal qualities when consciousness expands to include realization of other dimensions and one's multi-dimensional reality. Healing energy radiates out of the physical body, influencing all encountering your energy field.

Energetics of the oil

The scent of Basil stimulates a need for action. It awakens long-forgotten desires to let them be realized. Its spicy nature feels impregnated with a rich, intense energy vibration.

The energy of Basil opens energy pathways and generates an amplified vibration of Spirit that flows down onto the earth plane. Energetically, it opens the sinus cavities and throat chakra so you can breathe a greater amount of life's essence deeply into the root chakra and produce a greater feeling of being firmly grounded. This grounded connection stimulates an exuberant desire to live life more fully and infused with spiritual joy.

Use Basil oil when you have made the decision to live each moment as consciously as possible. Increasing consciousness requires repeated affirmation of your intention to be totally responsible for every action and thought. You must accept and own that you create your reality, and acknowledge and assume responsibility for the effect you have on everything that comes into your energy field. At first, it feels overwhelming, but through acceptance and living life with the greatest amount of integrity, you realize that the responsibility sets you free. Spiritual purpose begins to direct your every thought and action. Basil's energy significantly aids you in making the conscious choice to be a co-creator.

Basil helps us awaken to our spiritual Self. However, facing our true Self and accepting that aspect is often very difficult because we often lack self-esteem and feel unworthy of receiving the energy. As we increase our love of all aspects of ourselves, we permit a greater amount of Soul energy into the physical. We recognize the baggage that limits the increase of our Soul light. Basil oil energy can potentially produce tremendous discomfort when we avoid aspects of ourselves or invalidate them as unworthy. Basil pushes us to recall the issues that contribute to low self-worth and self-limitation. It is necessary to acknowledge and embrace these issues to overcome their influence. Basil energy gives strong support while mastering your ability to embrace in love the challenges of life, and find a state of acceptance.

Basil helps new thoughts and concepts flow easily into your changing reality. Use Basil oil when consciously working to overcome being rigidly judgmental and controlling of how you believe life should be.

Basil is an oil for teachers of New Age thought and philosophy. Energetically, the oil helps those called for service begin to establish the new paradigms of living in a love-based reality. These teachers need to demonstrate new paradigms in a widely-comprehensible manner that teaches through love instead of fear. Lessons learned in love increase our compassionate understanding of the path humanity has chosen to experience—learning through fear the journey of duality. Fear has been instrumental in increasing the separation from Spirit, and fear is the bridge that needs to be crossed in order to return.

Basil oil's energy is beneficial when you are at a crossroads in life or going through a spiritual death. The energy generates comfort to those undergoing initiations. Basil oil gives support in overcoming depression, doubt, worry, anxiety, or facing an unknown cause of suffering. Basil oil provides an energy for trusting in spirit and renews our zest for life by inspiring great enthusiasm.

Basil is known as the royal herb and many cultures developed an enriched lore about its essence. It is often associated with fertility and death. Like Spirit, it inherently contains both evil and the sacred in a true unified state.

Using the oil for transformation

Use Basil oil on the gall bladder and liver meridians to energetically support the ability to become more responsible. The stomach meridian influences the digestion, and using the oil there promotes self-nourishment and supports self-trust. Clearing constrictions in the stomach meridian enhances the ability to relax. Over-thinking and fretting will calm, allowing the physical body to experience greater relaxation. Energizing the triple warmer meridian with Basil oil permits a greater assimilation of energy through all the organ systems, enabling you to deeply experience emotions through the heart chakra. When at a crossroads in life, use Basil oil to clear any obstructions of energy in the triple warmer meridian and releases old patterns blocking progress. Clearing the heart and pericardium meridians heightens the ability to assimilate greater amounts of love or light energy into the physical. The oil penetrates the armor that shields a person from fully experiencing unconditional love and vulnerability and you to experience more joy. Massaging the oil onto the lungs, front and back, and the lung meridian stimulates the release of stored grief, sorrow, and anxiety, and generates more oxygenation to nourish the organ systems of the body. Basil oil nourishes the kidney meridian to support being in the moment. Use the oil on both the bladder and kidney meridians to release unconscious fears and unresolved emotions that hinder your ability to love yourself.

Precautions

Do not use this oil on children or infants. Avoid using during pregnancy. Diabetics should be cautious of this oil. This oil can be slightly irritating to the skin and potentially sensitizing; keep exposure to sunlight at a minimum. Dilute 15-20 drops of oil in 2 ounces of base oil. Always check for a reaction.

BERGAMOT   *Citrus aurantium bergamia – Rutaceae*
Transformations

Key: Communication with the Unseen. Bergamot helps the personality surrender its need to be in control and allows the forces of grace, wisdom, compassion, trust, and acceptance to direct life instead of fear. The power of
grace transforms old thought patterns caused by despair and guilt into joy,
contentment, serenity, and wisdom. Awareness of and communication with
the Unseen Realm are established. Self-love increases when resistance to
other possibilities is released.

Growth and healing issues

Awareness of how attached we are to maintaining mass consciousness and
limitation leads to overcoming enslavement to the physical. Basil helps us
realize the magnitude of separation we have created from Spirit and
encourages the desire to return to wholeness. Negative thoughts, beliefs
and emotions that maintain this powerless state are transformed with
truth. Depression, confusion, non-acceptance, judgments, and other forms
of constrictions are released.

Energetic influences on the bodies and chakras

The heart chakra expands, enabling a deeper connection with Spiritual
love. The solar plexus aligns with the heart to overcome power and control
issues. The Soul infuses with the personality. Bergamot releases fear and
trauma from the cellular memory of the physical body. The mental body
becomes calmer and clearer.

Energetics of the oil

Bergamot is known as the bitter orange. Energetically, it acknowledges the
bitterness the Self feels when it realizes the magnitude of the separation it
has created from Spirit. This oil helps you surrender into the power of
Grace and let it influence your life.

The lore surrounding the Orange claims that it was a gift to Earth from
another race of Beings. The oil of the celestial fruit attunes to the Angelic

realm, thereby enabling you to recognize and establish communication with the guardian angels and other beings of light watching and helping your spiritual evolution. Using Bergamot oil the personality begins integrating with the consciousness of the Higher Self. Energetically the oil eases fear held in the physical body. Once self-limitation releases, it advocates the expansion into new realms of awareness.

Bergamot helps dispel negative thoughts held in the mental and emotional bodies, a quality of energy shared with other members of the citrus family. It has a very uplifting energy that allows a state of mental clarity and calms the emotions. Bergamot oil relieves depression and stress-related conditions through its refreshing and cheerful inspiring qualities. Energetically, it directly stimulates the mental body to release depressive patterns. Releasing depressive patterns lets creativity begin to flow and stimulates a need for expression. It frees energy constriction in the subtle bodies, thereby encouraging spiritual growth.

The green color of Bergamot oil opens and expands the heart chakra, expanding its energy and heightening the capacity to feel greater love. Bergamot helps to transmute the dense energy held in the solar plexus chakra, aligning it with the heart's desires. Blocks between these chakras diffuse, aligning and integrating the chakras' energies. The ego's need for control is diminished and infused with a greater amount of Soul energy.

Bergamot oil's energy aids the release of constraints that maintain states of density by helping you to honestly acknowledge the root cause of these issues. The cause is often non-acceptance of self, which generates a lack of self-love. Bergamot oil assists in the transformational process of rebirth, naturally renewing enthusiastic life energy when the heart and solar plexus align. Irritability arising during transitions can be calmed with the oil's energy. Energy is better assimilated through all the bodies, encouraging new responses towards change.

Bergamot's energy reduces the programmed tendency towards resistance, aiding the mental body in assimilating concepts supporting new realities. Physical body cells become rejuvenated with this new consciousness, infused with joy and contentment, slowing the aging process. Consequently, repressed feelings of grief and despair transform into feelings of serenity and wisdom. Energetically, the oil acts to vitalize the etheric hypothalamus, pineal, and pituitary glands increasing the physical body's vibratory frequency. Bergamot also stimulates the recognition of thought patterns instrumental in aging the physical body. Recognition and constant awareness help to reprogram the mind to rejuvenate the physical body. Expressing emotions instead of denying their existence shatters the illusion that growing old and decrepit exhibits maturity and wisdom.

Bergamot oil cools excessive heat in the body. The tremendous amounts of energy being absorbed in the body produce heat. Friction generates when the templates between the physical, etheric, or subtle bodies become misaligned or retain dense residue. The burning of old karma and beliefs that no longer serve a purpose also produce heat. When these beliefs are transmuted by grace, they create a sensation of heat radiating out of the physical body. Releasing cellular memory and patterns of disharmony often creates heat. Bergamot energetically stimulates the etheric thyroid to balance the body's thermostat. Depression and unworthy feelings unbalance the physical thyroid and contribute to weakening the etheric organ. Bergamot helps restore harmony to the thyroid gland and, by increasing love and self-confidence, maintains balance. Meditating with Bergamot oil inspires a desire to permit receiving the essence of joy through many new channels.

Bergamot oil is traditionally associated with fertility rites. The white flowers of orange blossoms are a symbol of the Virgin Mary and the fruit is a product of her chastity. Meditating with Bergamot oil often recalls memories of past lives during the Italian Renaissance and in sixteenth-century France, or memories of lives spent along the Ivory Coast of Africa.

Using the oil for transformation

Use on the heart and solar plexus chakras to align their etheric energy and infuse it into the physical body. Bergamot oil releases relationship stress, with others and with self. To stimulate this release, massage the oil on the back and front of the heart, the shoulder blades, and the front clavicle region. Bergamot oil clears the spleen meridian of cords draining your energy, which promotes an expanded awareness of reality. Use the oil on the gall bladder meridian to encourage a greater ability to allow life to flow through challenges.

Massage into the large intestine meridian to release tightly held belief patterns that hinder movement or change. Use the oil on both the heart and pericardium meridians to move through relationship issues. Bergamot oil is valued for its uplifting qualities and blends well with other oils. Use on the inner-wrists, inner-elbow, and behind the knees to release the stagnated energy of negativism that has a tendency to collect in those areas. Massage into the area above the kneecap to stimulate heart hormones. Use on the ankles to help open up the energy of joy for the physical body.

Meditate with the oil when feeling guilt over past actions to acquire insights as to why the situation was originally created, what the experience taught, and to take responsibility for creating the experiences and acknowledge their higher purpose in evolving the self. This promotes greater trust for surrendering into Spirit's wisdom. Divine surrender stimulates greater compassion, less judgment, and more acceptance, allowing past injustices to be resolved by grace, which automatically releases guilt's heavy burden.

The antiseptic properties of this oil lend it to many uses. Use it in soaps for a clean fresh feeling that also revitalize the etheric body. Bergamot's energy clears skin blemishes such as boils and acne. Often the root cause of acne and boils is festering anger directed inwards or a lack of self-love. The oil helps provide insight into both issues.

Precautions

Citrus oils often have a high concentration of pesticides. This oil can be slightly irritating to the skin. Dilute 15-20 drops of oil in 2 ounces of base oil, and check for a reaction. Bergamot can be photosensitizing.

BLACK PEPPER   *Piper nigrum – Piperaceae*
Transformations

Key: Overcoming worry and anxieties. Black Pepper helps the mental, emotional and physical bodies become more receptive to spiritual guidance. Developing discernment and increasing Spiritual acceptance overcomes repression, misplaced responsibility, and burdens that cause suffering and pain. New beliefs are aligned as old realities change, allowing greater love and understanding to be felt. We are then able to focus and direct our intent to manifest our spiritual and physical needs.

Growth and healing issues

Black Pepper creates a stronger bond with spirit that diminishes feelings of imprisonment caused from worry, lack, anxiety, and despair over challenging life experiences that make us feel powerless. These overwhelming feelings lessen when greater self-worth, resourcefulness, and discernment are realized. Black Pepper helps us recognize denial, allowing burdens to resolve through self-acceptance and compassion.

Energetic influences on the body and chakras

Black Pepper aids etheric digestion and eases the frustration and anger caused by the conflict of old and new beliefs, which lessens resistance to change. Physical stamina increases when the subtle bodies align. Energetically it reduces the overwhelming anxiety of third dimensional density by stimulating the courage to address fears pertaining to low self-worth. Black Pepper also assimilates a greater amount of Spirit into the physical, expanding the light body energy and physically grounding it.

Energetics of the oil

Black Pepper's scent is sharp and penetrating. Black Pepper oil's energy is similar to the sudden awareness of holding one's breath.

The energy of Black Pepper oil helps overcome feelings of constraint and reduce overwhelming anxieties. This is a good oil to use when focusing on what you want to manifest. Often despair over the inability to pay bills, the lack of fulfilling employment, and other such experiences contribute to this stress. Focusing on anxieties about the future will magnetize that reality and make it occur. Focusing your energy on what you desire releases the need to be a victim. The key to fulfilling your needs is to confront insidious unconscious beliefs—not being good enough, or not deserving what you want, unable to or incapable of supporting yourself, money is evil—that hinder your needs being met. Black Pepper helps you acknowledge these beliefs and learn the lesson behind them so you may change them. It encourages a healthy self-value and resourcefulness and develops the discernment that prevents installing or maintaining destructive beliefs.

Energetically, Black Pepper works on the spiritual level to digest the feelings of frustration and anger about yourself. It opens the etheric digestive tract, enabling easy alignment of new realities with old beliefs. It is a very motivating energy and can stimulate the mind, physical body, and emotions to attune with Spiritual guidance. Increased energy through each of the bodies helps overcome denial. Meditating with Black Pepper oil helps you to be more alert when requesting guidance from Spirit, allowing you to achieve deeper concentration and clearly focus your intention.

Repressed emotions and memories become unconscious patterns of behavior. Black Pepper will strengthen the physical body's alignment to the subtle bodies, releasing stagnated energy caused by denial of emotions. Through this alignment, the light body is expanded, allowing a greater amount of light to assimilate and be used by the physical body. Black Pepper opens up the sinus passages, allowing tears to flow, cleansing and releasing these burdens. Feelings of freedom come from this release, enabling you to experience greater compassion and acceptance of yourself.

Using the oil for transformation

Black Pepper rubbed into the soft tissue area above the breast and shoulder joint (clavicle) helps to release hurt feelings. This point feels very tender when feelings of hurt and ridicule are suppressed in the body. Using the oil on the bladder meridian helps you stop holding onto painful feelings. Black Pepper oil on the large intestine meridian along the arms helps energy, let go and move on from depression and hopelessness. Use Black Pepper to clear the crown chakra and brow chakras. Use when experiencing frontal headaches as this often signals colon distress caused by not letting go. Rubbing the oil on the brow and webbing of the thumb and index finger helps relieve headaches.

Massaging Black Pepper oil into the small intestine meridian helps to lessen feelings of being trapped into limiting life situations. Using Black Pepper on the kidney meridian will help you live in the moment and reduce anxiety of the future, promoting feelings of self-trust. To conquer excessive worry, use the oil on the stomach and spleen meridians. Use on the liver meridian to help develop the ability to make responsible decisions and carry them to fruition. Rubbing Black Pepper oil on the soles of the feet will give you a boost of physical energy.

Precautions

Do not use this oil on children or infants. This oil can be slightly irritating to the skin and potentially sensitizing. Dilute 15-20 drops of oil in 2 ounces of base oil and check for a reaction.

CAJEPUT   *Melaleuca cajeputi – Myrtaceae*

Transformations

Key: Realizing dysfunctional relationships. Male traits of control, domination, aggression and logic integrate with the feminine traits of receptivity, creativity, emotional sensitivity, and the intuitive nature for achieving greater balance and wholeness. Relationships are created and motivated by true spiritual love when each partner realizes they are responsible for fulfilling their own needs, releasing the need to have their partner act out what they are unable to express.

Growth and healing issues

Cajeput helps you recognize and overcome dysfunctional and abusive relationship patterns, enabling you to create healthier and more harmonious behaviors. Discovering the root causes of sexual issues stimulates self-nurturing, creativity, and sensuality. Men in confusion over their feminine aspects can gain more clarity and understanding of themselves.

Energetic influences on the bodies and chakras

Cajeput clears energy obstructions in the root, sacral, solar plexus, and heart chakras that hinder intimacy and the ability to emotionally connect with others. Aligning and opening the root, sacral, solar plexus and heart chakras stimulates greater self-expression and satisfaction. Sexual abuse violations are released from the cellular memory.

Energetics of the oil

Cajeput smells delightful sometimes and at other times, rank. Energetically, Cajeput heightens your awareness of feelings of reluctance and inertia around issues you do not want to acknowledge.

Cajeput helps you address dysfunctional relationship patterns. Use it for discovering and overcoming inappropriate or dysfunctional energy patterns that repeatedly occur in your relationships. These patterns may be formed in the womb, in childhood, or even in a past life. These patterns could be traits inherited from either parent. Introspection while using Cajeput strengthens the courage needed to examine the root causes of behaviors, helping you understand their lesson and end the cycle.

Cajeput helps recall repressed memories of sexual abuse in this life or from other lifetimes that are stored in the root and sacral chakras and that distort the womb and sexual organ's energies. Cajeput oil stimulates the release of cellular memories held in these organs, promoting healing. Sexual issues can distort and obstruct the energy coming into these chakras, hindering the development of healthy and fulfilling intimate relationships. Refusing to recognize the root causes of a sexual issue can also block the throat chakra, distort thyroid energy, and create feelings of low self-esteem. Cajeput transmutes these energies of low self-esteem by opening and aligning the root and sacral chakras with the throat chakra, enabling greater expression of the true Self on all dimensions. Aligning this energy with the heart chakra helps you experience the ecstasy of sensuality and sexual creativity. You can fully experience sexuality without fear and lovingly embrace the shame and guilt feelings surrounding your sexuality.

The energy of Cajeput helps women who have had hysterectomies realize the root cause of the disease. This is crucial: removing the physical body's organs does not solve the problem, because the etheric body's organs are still intact. Often the root issue behind dis-ease remains in the etheric body's organs, and can cause problems in other physical body organs. Discovery of the root cause helps to realign sexual energy into greater creative expression and embracing the cause can promote healing of the organ. Discovering causes before the energy is terribly distorted might prevent physical illness.

Cajeput oil is useful for men in confusion over their feminine aspects. Social conditioning often makes men incapable of acknowledging their feminine aspects. Their model of the world reinforces the notion that male dominating, aggressive, and left brain energy, is necessary to success. External accomplishment is often the only way for men to generate an increased self-esteem. Intense emotional interaction is confusing and often shuts them down. Tempering and balancing male energy with feminine energy is a more receptive and intuitive approach to life. The energetics of the Cajeput, combined with the focused intention to emotionally relate, will help men develop these qualities. With comfortable awareness they can permit life to flow instead of needing to direct and control it. Experiencing the joy of emotionally relating increases a man's ability to nourish his Self with Spirit. He can establish communication, leading to healthier loving relationships. A deep sense of true intimacy is felt when sharing his Spiritual essence.

Using the oil for transformation

Using Cajeput oil on the reflex points of the hands and feet helps open the throat. Massaging Cajeput on the throat, womb, and ovaries on the body allows the release of suppressed sexual issues. Cajeput oil massaged on the gallbladder meridian allows memories of abuse to release from the physical cellular memory. Cajeput massaged into the conception meridian alleviates obstructions causing menstrual disorders and pain in the genital and pelvic regions. Use the oil on the governing meridian to overcome impotence and frigidity.

Massaging the oil into the arm and lung meridians helps reduce anxiety and sorrow. Massaging the oil on the sacrum enables a person to recognize the support they do have in life. Using the oil on the heart meridian relieves feelings of sadness and self-doubt. On the pericardium meridian, using Cajeput will stimulate greater intimacy in sexual relationships. Applying the oil on the triple warmer meridian with the intent to release old relationship patterns allows new roles to develop in relationships. This meridian also helps to heal energy drains. Cajeput oil massaged into the bladder meridian helps you realize feelings and attitudes about sexuality.

Massage the oil into the reflex points of the thyroid and reproductive organs on the hands and feet. The reproductive reflex point on the back heel of each foot responds to deeply rubbing the oil into the area. Often this area will feel very tender. While elevating the feet and holding a heel in each hand, apply pressure in a circular motion and then reverse the direction. Visualize sending love up the legs, and focus the intent to embrace with love the issue being recalled.

Precautions

Do not use this oil on children or infants. Be suspicious of this oil's purity because it is often diluted with synthetics or less expensive constituents. This oil can be slightly irritating to the skin and potentially sensitizing. Dilute 15-20 drops of oil in 2 ounces of base oil and check for a reaction.

CALAMUS ROOT   *Acorus calamus var. angustatus – Labiatae*
Transformations

Key: Identifies Family Behavioral Patterns. Healing family patterns, one member can end the pattern, raising the consciousness of the whole family. New directions and foundations build healthier and more satisfying relationships. Learning to love and honor your self encourages relationships that are nurturing and supportive.

Growth and healing issues

Helps us recognize inherited family patterns. Introspection into role models and the dynamics and behaviors of the family helps to overcome dysfunctional relationships. Family insights may also help find the causes of low self-worth, obsessive behavior, victim or abuser attitudes, and defensive reactions.

Energetic influences on the bodies and chakras

Releasing the stress of conflict in relationship patterns calms the nervous system. Improving communication between the emotional, mental, and physical bodies supports spiritual growth.

Energetics of the oil

The scent of Calamus Root is very pungent. The energy feels comforting and repulsive, quite similar to the feelings you may have about your family. Calamus is also known as sweet flag, a semi-aquatic reed plant with rhizomes that grow in mud. The rhizome root of Calamus is a symbolic representation of family genealogy, and the aquatic aspect symbolizes the collective emotional body of a family.

Calamus Root's scent helps bring to the surface genetically-imprinted family patterns that create energy distortions in emotional relationships. Family patterns often repeat through generations because the family never established a model or foundation for functional behavior. Inherited family dynamics create dysfunctional models for relationships with others and with self. Perpetual repetition of patterns underlies the vicious cycle of a victim becoming an abuser.

Calamus Root energy soothes intense emotions produced by dysfunctional relating skills. Healing begins when you choose not to continue the cycle and stop playing the family game. You can end any game by "taking your toys away"—learning another response. You must consciously define and create pictures of a healthy, supportive, and growth producing relationship. Affirming and clearly visualizing new behavioral models allows you to establish new responses. On an energetic level, this process can bring closure to a pattern and heal members of a family through many generations, raising the spiritual consciousness of the whole family. Only one family member needs to learn the lesson of the experience to end the pattern. When you quit the game, the other participant has no one to play with and must change.

Calamus Root eases obsessive behaviors based in low self-esteem and insecurity. Calamus Root allows you to look at behavior in a calmer state and from a different perspective, releasing the need for engaging a defensive reaction. Objective acknowledgement—honestly looking at ingrained beliefs without blame or rationalizing the behavior—lets lessons be learned and allows a greater sense of self-value by embracing into love judgments of unworthiness. Learning the lesson's purpose resolves resistance and the need to repeat the energy. Visualizing new reactions actualizes the reinforcement of a new behavior motivated by love. An obsession is resolved when new attitudes allow different responses to the energy.

Family "hooks" often attach into the spleen and distort its energy, which can cause you to feel tired and drained by family interaction. You can release the hooks in a meditation known as Shamanic cord releasing. Feel the energy in your body and visualize where you are attached to family and cut the cord or pull the hook out. Remember to pull your hooks out of the other person as well. Detaching the psychic bond contributes to healing family issues and re-balancing your spleen energy. Balanced spleen energy allows the mental body to become more receptive to communication from the emotional body. It frees the physical body of any need to exhibit chronic pain. Anxiety and internal struggles resolve by learning to relax and trust the life process.

Using the oil for transformation

Cajeput oil used on the triple warmer meridian enhances the ability to feel and experience warm family ties and helps overcome dysfunctional relationship patterns.

Using the oil on the heart and pericardium meridians will release energy obstructions that produce frigidity or a lack of intimacy in life. Opening heart and pericardium energy will release the tension and strife that come from closing off from the human desire for love. Choosing to focus on more appropriate models of healthy relationships will help to instill them into your life. This allows you to relax into intimacy unafraid. Using the oil on these meridians also promotes a greater sense of self-worth and self-esteem. It stimulates intimate relationships with self and others.

Calamus Root oil used on the governing meridian calms the nervous system, releasing unconscious death wishes and terror of living in the physical. It generates a greater ability to discern truth and promotes making conscious choices instead of reacting.

Unblocking the small intestine energy releases fragments of self lodged there, influencing low self-esteem and low self-value. To promote the ability to feel at ease with your self, use Calamus Root oil on the stomach, spleen, and gall bladder meridians. Using the oil on the liver meridian can transmute issues caused from anger and power abuses. Massage the oil onto the spleen area of the body to seal off energy drains from inappropriate family hooks.

Precautions

This oil can be internally toxic and potentially lethal. Be cautious when using it externally. Do not use this oil on children or infants.

CAMPHOR OF BORNEO

Dryobalanops aromatica / camphora – Dipterocarpeae

Transformations

Key: Uplifts Burdens. Calming the passions brings detachment from charged emotions, allowing greater clarity and objectivity to prevail. Increasing acceptance of other's differences and honoring everyone's path choice helps one become more responsible to self. Validating intuition permits the mental body to trust intuited information, regarding it as valuable and as accurate as logic thought.

Growth and healing issues

Helps to shatter the crystallization around deeply repressed beliefs held by the personality. Overcoming this resistance encourages introspection into relationship patterns, sexual issues, and intense denial. Helps us understand that we have misplaced our sense of duty and responsibility in the ego instead of Spirit.

Energetic influences on the bodies and chakras

Establishes communication and integration between the unconscious and conscious minds, which helps to bypass mind filters, judgments, and attitudes. Messages from the Higher Self are more readily received and acted upon. Dialogue with each of the bodies promotes greater acceptance between them and reduces internal conflict.

Energetics of the oil

Camphor of Borneo's sharp and penetrating scent awakens a feeling of forgetting something. Its energy dissolves crystallized, ingrained beliefs that change is unattainable. Camphor of Borneo lightens mental, emotional, and spiritual burdens.

Camphor of Borneo oil calms the passions and disengages you from charged emotions. Disconnecting from the intensity attached to emotions results in a more objective point of view supporting recognition of how your actions create situations. With this insight you can take responsibility for your part and change the situation if you so desire. Responsibility means to respond to what makes your heart sing as opposed to the burden of duty.

Camphor of Borneo oil helps us realize each individual must live their life and learn their own unique lessons. It is important not to be invested in another's reactions. They are reacting according to their own fears and judgments. It is best to see and hold an individual in the thought of love and perceive their magnificence, not their personality. Affirm that it is all right for them to be on their path, this furthers your own acceptance of what is in your highest good.

Camphor oil opens up a direct link between the unconscious and conscious minds. This link can bypass the logical mind so messages from Spirit are more readily accepted. The emotional body's ability to feel allows interpretation of abstract messages from subtle energies. Intuition—interpreting messages from dreams, nature, body reactions, and other sources—is often hindered when the logical minds acts as a strong filter disclaiming or invalidating the information. The mental body knows how to survive painful experiences through conditioning and often establishes its conditioning as the way. The mental body takes control, perpetuating rigidity. Through persistent vigilance this defense mechanism can be trained to rely on intuition. The training process requires attentive acknowledgment of all intuitive flashes. Take note of each occurrence and the subtle manner in which the message was perceived. This validates intuition and mentally reinforces its accuracy. Gradually the mental body will begin to trust the emotional and physical bodies' intuitive reasoning. Establishing dialogue between each of the bodies permits them to work together in a harmonious integrated manner.

Camphor of Borneo oil helps to alleviate the symptoms of migraine headaches. Migraines frequently come from resistance between the mental, emotional, and spiritual bodies. A collision between spirit and matter accurately describes the intensity of these headaches. Pain in the physical body is also created from resistance to change, not being validated, or needs not being met.

Using the oil for transformation

Use on the lung meridian to allow deeper breathing and open the sinus passages. Massaging Camphor oil deeply into the arms releases blocked energy that might induce headaches. Using Camphor oil on the gallbladder and liver meridians also provides relief for headache symptoms. Use Camphor oil on the bladder meridian to release suppressed feelings. Massaging Camphor oil into the spleen helps to balance and energize energy in the body. Applying Camphor oil aligns spiritual energy with the heart, the third eye, and the crown chakras. Camphor combined with other essential oils enhances the energetic qualities of the oils.

Precautions

Avoid using during pregnancy. Be suspicious of this oil's purity as it is often diluted with synthetics or less expensive constituents. This oil could be problematic for people who suffer with allergy and asthma. This oil can be slightly irritating to the skin and potentially sensitizing. Dilute 15-20 drops of oil in 2 ounces of base oil and check for a reaction.

Camphor of Borneo is not related to the toxic camphor that is an ingredient in mothballs. Toxic camphor is not used in aromatherapy. Camphor oil works against the effectiveness of homeopathic remedies.

CARDAMON SEED   *Elettaria cardamonum – Zingiberaceae*
Transformations

Key: Enhances Assimilation of Energy. Emotional balance is achieved and maintained by learning to be motivated by love and compassion. This allows new energies and more light to be gently assimilated into the physical body. We then begin to recognize true spiritual love for ourselves and others.

Growth and healing issues

Achieves an easier acceptance of new thoughts and beliefs that are contrary to the mass consciousness. Recognizes fears that close the heart chakra. Helps to distinguish the pain and suffering that a closed heart produces. Imparts the awareness of how we manipulate ourselves by using substitutions for love.

Energetic influences on the bodies and chakras

Various forms of stress caused from attachment to old beliefs and dogmatic, rigid attitudes, produce great resistance and internal conflict in the digestive region. Cardamon Seed oil aids in releasing these attachments and allowing calm to be felt. Cardamon helps maintain an open heart when experiencing fear. This frees energy constrictions in the body. Developing better communication between the bodies reduces the internal stress that causes disease.

Energetics of the oil

Cardamon Seed's exotic scent transports the mind to strange and colorful artists' marketplaces. Energetically, Cardamon oil allows new energies to assimilate gently into the physical body.

Cardamon Seed oil's energy benefits those individuals working on digesting new ideas and thoughts that are contrary to mass consciousness. The mental body believes that it needs to relate with mass consciousness thought patterns because they are the known path for survival. The conflict between a person's old reality system and new ideas and beliefs creates stress and increases the fear level in the mental body. Just the thought of change can create stress feelings in some people. Cardamom soothes heartburn, which arises from unadulterated fear that closes the heart chakra.

Many instinctive survival memories are stored in the digestion region. Using Cardamon Seed oil alleviates stress held in the digestion region, which in turn releases the rigid and dogmatic attitudes maintaining the stress. Conflicting realities are noticed in the colon and stomach as distress, a dense and heavy feeling. The physical body attempts to communicate to the mental body by creating distress in the physical body. Prolonged denial of these unresolved issues in the body can create cancerous conditions. Acknowledging and embracing the issue as a valid feeling and loving the issue promotes the healing process. Doing the embracing process facilitates the release of constraints in the body's energy flow and allows a greater amount of light to become available to heal the physical symptoms.

Cardamon is an antidote for sugar cravings. Sugar is an addictive substance that, because it is associated with treats, is used as a substitution for real heart love. Cardamon oil allows you to begin feeling the sweetness of life again through expanding the heart chakra. In addition it opens the energy of the etheric pancreas, which becomes blocked with over consumption of sugar. An unobstructed etheric pancreas allows emotional balance, greater compassion, and communicating from a place of love.

Cardamon is a widely used spice with ancient origins in India. Energetically, this oil stimulates memories of the collective consciousness of Hindu cultures and lifetimes in India. The Hindu Ayurvedic and Chinese systems of medicine have long used Cardamon for many medicinal purposes. The Egyptians used the spice in religious ceremonies, while the Arab caravans introduced the spice as a perfume into the Roman and Greek cultures.

Using the oil for transformation

Anointing the crown chakra, the very top of the head, helps connect the crown energy with the second sacral chakra and balances the energy flow between the chakras. Cardamon aids the digestion and stimulates the small and large intestine meridians to increase assimilating emotions and allow old patterns to release. Rubbing Cardamon into the belly or ovary areas of the sacral chakra grounds an individual.

Massaging the stomach meridian with the oil calms worry. Always massage the oil into the colon area in a right-to-left direction. The abdominal, solar plexus, and pancreas area all benefit from Cardamon Seed oil. Use the oil on the kidney meridian points on the back and legs to help calm mistrust, fear, or anxiety felt when you are working to develop new thought patterns. When experiencing a great amount of fear use the oil on the kidney and bladder meridian points to help restore a sense of peace. Just close your eyes and inhale this warm exotic scent for an uplifting experience.

Precautions

This oil is fairly non-irritating, to be certain check for a reaction. Use 15-30 drops in 2 ounces of a base oil.

CARROT SEED   *Daucus carota – Umbelliferae*
Transformations

Key: Expands and Grounds Consciousness. Control becomes unnecessary when we realize it is a form of self-limitation. Greater self-acceptance stimulates compassion and joy. Integrating Soul energy with the personality's male and female qualities manifests as creative power. True purpose and meaning for conceiving life on all dimensions are realized; along with responsibility for one's creations. A greater alignment with Spirit increases the power of our thoughts.

Growth and healing issues

Clarity and knowledge heightens on the journey of self-discovery. Wisdom increases, enabling simultaneous multi-dimensional and physical grounding. Illuminates the realization that the mind has the power and ability to be either constructive or destructive.

Energetic influences on the body and chakras

More Spiritual energy becomes grounded into the physical. The third eye opens, expands and connects with the root chakra for clearer inner vision, producing a more realistic and healthier view of self.

Energetics of the oil

Inhaling Carrot Seed oil creates a feeling of calmness and surety of knowing. It creates clarity of inner vision and heightens perception to assist you on the journey of self-discovery. Energetically, it empowers a grounded view of self by opening the third eye and connecting the energy into the root chakra. Great wisdom is initiated with this oil. Some of that wisdom generates the ability to be simultaneously multidimensional and grounded into the physical. No small feat!

Energetically the oil awakens the ability to understand another person's point of view, thus increasing our compassion for understanding the struggles and joys each individual creates for achieving Spiritual evolution. This understanding also promotes greater acceptance of self, releasing judgments and the need to control life. This expanded perception is an opportunity for Spirit to begin the process of integrating with the personality.

The inherent characteristics of Carrot Seed oil create the feeling of being solidly grounded. Carrot Seed helps in overcoming fear of defeat by recognizing the lesson experienced. It creates an understanding of the

meaning of balance and wholeness. The oil energetically integrates masculine and feminine qualities of the Soul with the personality's energy, creating balance by tempering the masculine aggressive power with the feminine passive creativity.

Often this energy brings into awareness sexual issues that arise from
misunderstanding male and female energies. The Soul's true united state is
androgynous; the personality evolves by manifesting the Soul's balanced
male and female qualities. This union awakens an understanding of the true
purpose of the conflict of duality: through such an understanding, the
experience of Oneness may be realized.

Carrot Seed teaches us to be aware the effects our actions and thoughts
have on other dimensions, and the accountability that we incur. To become
truly conscious realized beings we must take full responsibly for the consequences our actions and thoughts have on all life in all dimensions and the
probabilities they set in motion. We do not realize how powerful our
thoughts are and the unintentional havoc they can produce.

It is important to note here that constant daydreaming, obsessing, fantasizing, or dwelling on a particular individual without their permission is an
infringement on their energy. Though unintentional, this is a psychic attack.
Budding romantic relationships best illustrate this. For example, you go out
on a date with someone and have a good time, exchanging phone numbers
for future contact. Then you begin constantly fantasizing about them and creating expectations, awaiting the Big Phone Call. The object of this projected
energy might not consciously know you are the cause of this bombardment
of energy. But they will unconsciously feel it and intuitively perceive that you
have a smothering, jealous, possessive, clinging, or overwhelming energy.
Not that anything happened on the physical plane to suggest this type of
energy but they will assuredly feel it. Hence, no call. Think before you think
too much—you are responsible for all aspects of your actions and thoughts.

Becoming more aligned with Spirit increases the power of our thought.
Taking conscious responsibility increases the Spiritual light channeled into the

physical body and along with that is the realization that it influences everything animate and inanimate. It raises the vibratory frequency in you and everything that your aura encounters. You need to be aware that not everyone accepts or is able to feel harmonious with this increased energy. Often they are unable to stay very long in the vibration and if they do they will unconsciously need to initiate some type of conflict to resonate with their density.

Carrot Seed oil grounds a great amount of Spiritual energy into the physical plane. People facilitating healing body work benefit by using the oil to channel greater amounts of Spiritual energy. Carrot Seed oil helps you realize the true meaning and purpose for conceiving life on all dimensions. Use Carrot Seed oil in meditation when deciding to have children. Massaging on the conception vessel meridian also helps dissolve the fears a potential mother might have about birthing a child and the terror felt from being on the earth plane. If a mother examines her fears of being here on the Earth plane, she will not readily pass them onto her child.

Using the oil for transformation

Using Carrot Seed oil on the spleen meridian helps to energize and balance the physical body. Energetically the oil promotes metabolism of vitamin A into the etheric body. The regenerative energy of the oil helps wounds heal faster. Carrot Seed seals energy leaks when massaged on the body. Using the oil on the kidney meridian increases vitality and growth. Rubbing the oil into the head points of the gallbladder and liver meridians releases frustration and allows greater harmony to flow.

Massaging the oil into the liver meridian helps to integrate the whole self by balancing the upper and lower body. Using the oil on the root and sacral chakras stimulates a grounded feeling. The reflex point on the inner hollow of the ankle also promotes grounding, and aligns the silver cord with the body—the dreaming body lifeline. Carrot Seed oil generates courage to face reality shifts by aligning the energy of the third eye with the first chakra—massage the oil on the forehead and temples to open and balance the third eye chakra and massage the oil into the governing meridian to release any obstructions. Using the oil on the triple warmer meridian stimulates the pituitary gland and aids in opening the third eye.

Precautions

Avoid using during pregnancy. Carrot Seed oil is fairly non-irritating, to be certain check for a reaction. Use 15-30 drops in 2 ounces of a base oil.

CEDAR LEAF (CEDARWOOD, THUJA)

Cedrus atlantica Manetti – Pinaceae

Transformations

Key: Comprehension of Spiritual Love. Spiritual love stimulates feelings of being totally secure and protected. Working to achieve greater clarity and direction of focus encourages discovering your true reality. Cedar oil generates greater self-acceptance and self-love.

Growth and healing issues

Helps to generate the hope and faith needed to achieve what the heart desires. Illuminates and identifies the difference between lust and love and fantasy projections of love. Also dispels the illusion of looking for love.

Energetic influences on the body and chakras

Cedar releases energy constrictions, allowing all the bodies to be nourished and balanced by a steady flow of energy. The heart chakra of the mental body aligns with the physical to reveal the difference between fantasy projections and true spiritual love.

Energetics of the oil

The scent of Cedar evokes an image of a room containing many doors. You know that one of the doors opens into the passageway leading to your heart's desire. The Cedar family of oils stimulates the hope and faith you need to choose the magical door. Cedar oil stimulates memories of feeling true Spiritual love and generates feelings of being totally secure and protected by that love.

Cedar's beneficial energy dispels the illusions surrounding the search for love and can restore lost faith to those searching. In reality we don't need to search for love. True love just is! There are no strings or commitments to true love. It is the substance of creation, and we often forget it is the same stuff that we are made of. To find love we only need to reconnect into it.

Cedar helps us get back in touch with our true reality by affirming and clarifying our focus. We learn to honestly identify the fantasy projections our minds have created about what love is. Once the illusions of romance and lust are separated from the source of true love, we more clearly feel and recognize the love within our hearts. A union between two people can be a wondrous experience that supports and teaches tremendous spiritual growth, but it is important to comprehend that the love comes from within each individual's Spiritual essence, not from the union. This love can never be lost.

Working with Cedar oil brings up issues that have doused the heart's fire. Accepting all aspects of self returns us to that place where true love is generated. Love must first be kindled within before it can truly burn outward. Cedar aligns the heart chakra of the mental body to the physical and allows the experience of just being.

Cedar brings the subtle bodies into balance by opening up any energy constrictions and enabling a steady flow of energy throughout all the bodies. It has a purifying energy that helps to release emotional toxins lodged in the subtle bodies. Cedar releases stress and anxiety from the mental and physical body. Energetically Cedar focuses mental energy and maintains a balance against the confusion caused by too many ideas coming into sudden awareness. Inhaling Cedar relaxes an over-analytic mind. Use Cedar before and after business meetings to generate greater clarity, to quickly perceive the core issue, or to get to the point.

Bible verses praised the sacred Cedars of Lebanon. It was widely believed that Cedar trees embodied a protective charm that drove away evil demons. The Cedar groves had the same status as the Druids' Oak trees. They were believed to be sacred oracles that communicated with those entrusted with ability to interpret their messages.

Using the oil for transformation

Cedar oil on the kidney meridian helps with issues of fear and mistrust that hinder the ability to love. Using Cedar oil on the triple warmer meridian helps overcome old patterns and fantasies about love. To generate a greater ability to feel protected through self-nourishment, use the oil on the pericardium meridian. This releases any blockages constricting the energy flow. Use Cedar oil on the heart meridian to enable a greater enjoyment of self by releasing the need for substitutes for love. Energetically opening the heart channel will also release the anxiety of needing to fill the void, creating a space to initiate knowing and recognizing more aspects of the self. Rubbing Cedar oil on the front and back of the heart chakra feels very nourishing to the physical body.

Using Cedar oil on the large intestine meridian will promote letting go and make it easier to flow with change. Clearing restrictions in the liver meridian harmonizes emotions and initiates a clearer view of the choices made in life and an ability to act with a greater sense of responsibility. Massaging the liver and gallbladder meridians' promotes the release of physical toxins in the body. Energizing the liver meridian with the oil allows a greater integration of the whole self.

Precautions

If you have epilepsy, be careful of both inhaling and using Cedar externally. If high blood pressure is present Cedar oil can be used cautiously in baths and highly diluted as a massage oil, but not inhaled. Do not use this oil on children or infants. Avoid using during pregnancy. This oil could be problematic for people who suffer with allergies and asthma. Cedar oil is often diluted with turpentine. Cedar oil can irritate the skin and mucous membranes. Dilute 1-10 drops in 2 ounces of a base oil before applying to the skin. Use only 1-5 drops in a bath.

CELERY SEED   *Apium graveolens – Umbelliferae*

Transformations

Key: Develops Tenderness. Stimulates insights about the role of fatherhood and illuminates the root cause of fatherhood issues. Helps resolve the feelings of being burdened by duty, the need to control, and the responsibility of providing the families physical needs. Celery Seed is especially helpful to those seeking to overcome identifying and valuing themselves only by their material success.

Growth and healing issues

Celery Seed awakens tenderness in the heart, altering a rigid and coldly detached personality. Allows recognition of the moodiness and nervousness caused by feelings of hurt and vulnerability.

Energetic influences on the bodies and chakras

Celery Seed balances the sodium and sugar levels of the etheric body and allows the etheric heart to function correctly. People feel their heart chakras begin expanding and come into balance. Celery Seed oil's calming energy eases moodiness.

Energetics of the oil

Notice how celery stalks surround the soft inner heart of the plant. The energetics of Celery Seed oil heightens the awareness of the rigid outer personality to the heart's inner tenderness. Celery Seed oil aligns heart energy with Spiritual purpose.

The energy of Celery acts as an emotional diuretic, releasing slights and hurts held in the mental and the emotional bodies. Celery oil soothes nervousness. Celery Seed oil can calm the moodiness that comes at that time of the full moon. Celery Seed oil balances the sodium in the etheric body, enabling the heart to function correctly. Celery also contributes to balancing blood sugar problems in the etheric body.

Celery oil softens the masculine matter-of-fact or cold mercurial attitudes. Celery seed can open and balance masculinity in the heart chakra. Its energy releases the rigidity of masculine emotional behavior conditioned for interacting with society. It mellows the consciousness that builds rigid walls.

Often, men who lost their fathers early in life were required to fill the male role in the family. They learned to sacrifice their playful childhood to the burdensome roles of provider and protector. Young women also took on the sole support of the family. These young adults grew up too fast taking care of their families' emotional and monetary needs. The overwhelming focus on others' needs deprived them of the time and focus to develop their spiritual identity. Using Celery oil encourages releasing the burdens and beliefs of duty and feelings of grief they might have unconsciously developed. Celery Oil promotes the ability to let go of the need to control and begin living life on their terms. They learn to relax into life and feel a deeper sense of joy and freedom.

A perfect time to use Celery Oil is when you have decided to start a family. Celery Oil allows you to explore what the role of fatherhood truly means to you. Meditate with the oil to review repressed issues that might arise with parenthood. You can use Celery oil to examine your own relationship with your father. Celery oil is helpful for women seeking to discover their unconscious beliefs and expectations about the role of fatherhood before they project them on their husbands.

Using the oil for transformation

The energy of Celery Seed oil stimulates the root chakra. Massage it along the spine, running the energy from the base up into the back heart chakra. Rub on the spleen meridian to clear issues of the nuclear family or issues dealing with family blood ties. Celery helps to seal the spleen energy against outside influences when draining family bonds are present. Rubbing the oil into the heart and triple warmer meridians helps you experience warmer emotional feelings from family and social interaction. Use on the spleen meridian also helps overcome worry and suppressed feelings of hurt.

Using Celery Oil on the liver meridian will help to release the guilt and anger produced by the burden of responsibility and allows you to acquire better responses to life. Massaging the oil on the bladder meridian releases feelings of burden and relaxes tightness felt in the shoulder region. Massaging Celery oil into the lung meridian helps release grief and sorrow and overcomes feelings of loss.

Precautions

Avoid using during pregnancy. Check for a reaction. Use 15-30 drops in 2 ounces of a base oil. Celery Seed oil can be photosensitizing; keep exposure to sunlight at a minimum.

CHAMOMILE   *Chamaemelum nobile:Matricaria chamomilla/recutita – Compositae*

Transformations

Key: Instills the Wisdom of Peace. Calming the conscious mind overcomes the need to be in control, allowing greater receptivity of intuitive messages. Chamomile heightens trance channeling and communication with the Higher Self. This promotes reception of spiritual will and spiritual purpose to guide the personality.

Growth and healing issues

Chamomile Oil promotes feeling at peace with your self, generating more self-love and transforming feelings of self-disgust, anger, loneliness, abandonment, and grief. The development of patience and self-nurturing helps you live in Divine Right Timing. Shifting this energy promotes greater communication with the Angelic Realm, heightens telepathic skills and allows easier energy transitions to be experienced.

Energetic influences on the bodies and chakras

The energy of Chamomile sedates the nervous system, calming the stress lodged in the mental, emotional, and physical bodies. Stress releases when the physical and subtle bodies align with the wisdom of peace. Releasing anger and subtle death wishes expands and rejuvenates the etheric liver. Heartbreak and the feeling of lost love are soothed by this expanded vibrational field.

Energetics of the oil

Chamomile feels like a Grandmother's gentle loving embrace. Chamomile oil balances the energy between Spirit and matter. Using Chamomile also transmutes feelings of self-disgust into nurturing feelings of self-love.

Energetically, Chamomile has an inherent sedating quality that can be useful to enhance trance channeling. The energy relaxes the conscious mind's need to be in control, thus promoting acceptance of intuitive messages. Meditating with Chamomile oil strengthens receptivity to Spiritual will and Spiritual purpose. Chamomile oil helps you develop patience and incur understanding about the order of Divine Right Timing. Chamomile is an excellent oil to use in conjunction with regression therapies because it supports a calm remembrance of otherwise intense experiences.

On the physical level, Chamomile acts on the nervous system. It has a deeply sedative action and can be euphoric. It also relieves inflammation caused by holding onto beliefs that no longer work in your present reality and must be released. Chamomile Oil expands the subtle etheric liver by releasing stored anger and death wishes originating through separation from Source. Separation creates feelings of loneliness and the longing to be some place other than in the moment. Returning to Source rejuvenates the etheric liver and begins to detoxify the physical body. The many toxic emotions arising from issues held in each organ's cellular memory gently begin to release, nourishing the physical organs.

The energy of Chamomile comforts feelings of abandonment. It can be a soothing balm for grief over the loss of a loved one and is a wonderful and consoling oil to use during the mourning period. Chamomile oil feels soothing to those making life transitions by alleviating the fears surrounding death. It helps you to comprehend the truth about immortality.

Chamomile oil provides assistance to earth-bound beings afraid of going into the light. If you feel the presence of a ghost, use Chamomile oil to create a vibratory field of love around the deceased spirit. Calling upon the Angelic Realm to help open the tunnel of light will help the Spirit make the transformation.

Chamomile oil generates understanding of Divine Grace at an emotional level. Chamomile opens the capacity for receiving intuition, thus reinforcing a deeper connection with Source. It also enhances the ability to feel and hear the Angelic Realms. Chamomile promotes communication between the realms and heightens telepathic skills. Use Chamomile oil in meditation when calling on the Angelic realm and feel the results.

Using the oil for transformation

The body craves Chamomile, which is why it is used in many body care products. Chamomile oil rubbed on the stomach and liver area feels wonderfully nurturing. Anointing the jawbone with Chamomile gently releases anger. Using Chamomile oil on the large intestine meridian helps to overcome self-judgment and induces the ability to let go. Chamomile oil massaged into the conception meridian helps overcome the terror of being separated from Source. Massaging the oil into the governing meridian overcomes the fear of living and dying.

Chamomile on the stomach meridian promotes self-acceptance and self-nurturing. Using Chamomile oil on the heart and pericardium meridians generates feelings of protection by increasing self-value and self-esteem. The heart and throat embrace the nourishment provided by Chamomile oil. Use the oil on the forehead and neck to calm and release tension felt in the head. Ease heartaches by massaging the oil into the thymus and heart area. Use Chamomile in massage for nourishing and soothing the nervous system.

Precautions

Chamomile is fairly non-irritating, to be certain check for a reaction. Use 15-30 drops in 2 ounces of a base oil.

CINNAMON   *Cinnamonum zeylanicum /*
                                         Cinnamonum cassia — Lauraceae

Transformations

Key: Awareness of Enslavement. Attitudes that support enslavement transform into abundance and freedom. Karma created in past lives resolves, permitting consciousness to shift its focus for gaining a greater awareness of a reaction's root cause.

Growth and healing issues

Cinnamon stimulates a need to recognize what things, beliefs, patterns, and attachments are creating enslavement and limitation. It brings the root causes of anger and abusive behavior to the surface and promotes greater conscious awareness about what emotions are being held and in what part of the body.

Energetic influences on the bodies and chakras

Cinnamon releases abuse, anger, rage, frustration and traumatic emotions programmed into the cellular memory. It helps to maintain a balanced energy when going through transitions. Cinnamon allows energy to flow unimpeded through the physical and subtle bodies.

Energetics of the oil

Cinnamon feels like a hot fireball of energy freeing and purifying everything in its path. It energetically works to free the memories of enslavement held deep in the unconscious. Often these memories have developed from lifetimes of victim behavioral patterns repressed in the unconscious mind. These unresolved memories produce the patterns that create enslavement to jobs, relationships, or families. Enslavement also comes from dogmatic attachment to convictions. Cinnamon oil works to overcome and transform the enslavement mentality into the true state of abundance. It also assists to remember the grief or comprehend the reasons for your rebellious nature and distaste for authority that derive from lifetimes of being a slave, indentured servant, or powerless. The oils can help to generate insights into the reasons that you give away your power or resist taking control of your power, and not feeling empowered or able to empower others.

Absence of happiness in life and work signals that energy is out of balance and suggests a need to shift the focus of consciousness. True freedom comes from releasing the limitation caused by entrenched thought patterns. Energetically, Cinnamon oil lifts up the mental body for seeing different perspectives. Cinnamon oil helps you overcome passionate convictions attached to emotionally charged situations. Cinnamon's energy generates new attitudes and allows you to feel and respond differently in challenging situations, enabling a greater realm of possibilities. Enlarging your view of the world creates an enhanced feeling of balance, especially when moving through changes.

Energetically, Cinnamon oil releases anger held in the cellular memory of the body and is an important oil to use when healing the scars of physical abuse in this life or past lives. Sometimes when memories of abuse start to release, the physical body might suddenly display the original scars of being beaten or whipped. The oil is powerful and can begin releasing in a manner similar to the original cause. When using Cinnamon oil, remind the body that it exists in the present so that it will help to release memories of abuse in a gentler manner. Cinnamon energy helps the body begin discharging energy distortions caused by repressed rage, frustration, and other limiting emotions held in the cellular memory. Cinnamon works directly on moving blocked energy out of the physical and etheric bodies. Cinnamon assists with honest introspection into the causes of emotional reactions and promotes overcoming the issues.

Historically, Cinnamon was a form of currency much like salt was. This coveted spice was a motivating force behind the creation of new trade routes. Energetically, Cinnamon oil also produces a motivating energy within the body. Many Chinese herbal remedies use Cinnamon because of its effectiveness in increasing the circulation. It has powerful anti-viral properties that many people relied upon to ward off plagues during Biblical times. Ancient Egyptian embalming practices preserved the body with Cinnamon oil.

Using the oil for transformation

Massage Cinnamon oil into the root chakra for a grounded and revitalized feeling. A closed root chakra disconnects you from feeling life's vitality. Opening the root chakra generates deeper feelings of physical life, which encourages the will to live.

A cup of sea salt added to a bath with a few drops of Cinnamon oil enhances the healing of the raw emotions around abuse. A Cinnamon oil bath also helps release anger and other constricting emotions. Constriction in energy circulation happens when the heart closes down to feeling, creating a weak heart connection with life. Using the oil on the heart meridian provides the means to cope with change. Use on the lung meridian supports the ability to let go and let be.

Massaging the oil into the pericardium meridian supports feelings of intimacy and enhances security with self. Using Cinnamon on the triple warmer meridian releases old relationship patterns and allows new bonds to be forged. Cinnamon on the small intestine meridian allows feelings of being trapped in relationship patterns to release. Massaging Cinnamon oil on the kidney meridian helps to overcome mistrust, fear, and anxiety, thus helping you live more in the present moment.

Precautions

Cinnamon oil can irritate the skin and mucous membranes. Dilute 1-10 drops in 2 ounces of a base oil and check for a reaction before applying to the skin. Use only 1-5 drops in a bath. Do not use this oil on children or infants.

CITRONELLA   *Cymbopogon nardus – Gramineae*
Transformations

Key: Calms Quick Anger. Citronella energy lends comfort and courage to confront and resolve conflicts present in one's life. Pesky irritations are overcome by having greater acceptance.

Growth and healing issues

Citronella acknowledges the frustrations that contribute to caustic speech and uplifts pessimistic emotions that shade a person's outlook and motivation, promoting a change in attitude. The scent is a natural bug deterrent, which allows a more joyful experience of nature.

Energetic influences on the bodies and chakras

Calming anger energetically soothes the nervous system. Learning to confront and express anger and frustration in a constructive manner raises vibrational frequency.

Energetics of the oil

Citronella's scent recalls fond memories of outdoor activities. Quick flaring anger is calmed by Citronella. Citronella calms eruptions over the small pesky things in life and supports examining the causes of these eruptions to find the deeper underlying issue. Citronella repels mosquitoes, which are attracted to anger in a person's energy field.

A sugar imbalance in the body system also attracts mosquitoes. Attraction to sugar may stem from the feelings that life has lost its joy. Feelings of anger or frustration may create an overwhelming craving for sweets. Excessive sugar consumption contributes to an irritable disposition. Overloading the adrenaline glands with sugar consumption engages the "fight or flight" syndrome of the sympathetic nervous system. Citronella oil energetically soothes the nervous system.

Citronella oil helps people who avoid conflict by generating a steady calm energy for approaching the confrontation. Use in meditation when dealing with confrontation to align with your Higher Self and call in the other person's Higher Self to resolve the matter with love. Doing this meditation before a physical confrontation prepares the personalities to be less combative.

Citronella also helps those prone to using caustic speech. Citronella influences the mental body, transmuting frustration out of the throat chakra and allowing calmer feelings to be expressed through speech.

Citronella uplifts pessimistic attitudes, encouraging different attitudes and courses of action. Citronella mixed with other oils enhances and magnifies the synergy of the blend.

Using the oil for transformation

Warming Citronella oil in an aromatherapy lamp refreshes a room and keeps bugs away and clears residues of anger and irritability vibrating in the space. Citronella oil's antiseptic properties have a cleansing effect. Using Citronella oil in a bath or a massage lotion releases feelings of uncleanness and shame. Citronella oil can clear skin eruptions such as pimples and acne, the root cause for skin outbreaks often being irritation with your self. Using the oil on the liver, large intestine, and spleen meridians calms feelings of anger. The oil massaged into the stomach meridian helps to overcome feelings of rebellion and anti-social behaviors. Open the throat by massaging Citronella oil into the lung, conception, and heart meridians. Massage Citronella oil into the stomach, gall bladder, and kidney meridians to uplift pessimism and bring more joy into life.

Precautions

Citronella oil is fairly non-irritating; to be certain check for a reaction. Use 15-30 drops in 2 ounces of a base oil.

CLARY SAGE   *Salvia sclarea – Labiatae*
Transformations

Key: Cleanses and Energizes the Mental Body. Stops constant mind chatter, which allows experiencing the stillness of joy. The mental and emotional bodies align with Spirit to better actualize Spirit into action. Calming and expanding the mental body's focus allows for greater clarity and to achieve being fully present and conscious in the moment.

Growth and healing issues

Clary Sage oil stills the mind's chatter, reducing confusion. It reduces paranoia and obsessive thought patterns that produce great resistance towards change, and lightens the dense energy of depression, sorrow, and fear that create barriers between personality and Spirit.

Energetic influences on the bodies and chakras

Clary Sage releases the mental body's heavy burdens by transmuting the thought forms surrounding the aura that maintain mental confusion, deplete the energy field, and scatter your focus.

Energetics of the oil

To describe Clary Sage's energy, imagine running down a hill as fast as possible, flapping your arms into the wind, creating the sensation of flying. Clary Sage oil invokes a feeling of true, unencumbered joy.

Getting the mind out of the way supports feeling true joy. Dense mental thought patterns can create feelings of depression, sorrow, and fear and create a cloud of confusion around the auric body. It is necessary to routinely clear and clean emotional thought patterns out of the aura. When this energy builds up, it scatters the mental body's ability to focus and creates confusion and a feeling of being overwhelmed, and also leads to panic and anxiety attacks. This may contribute to creating a delusional reality.

Clary Sage oil's energy cleans the debris out of the mental body, calming the constant mind chatter. It helps the mental body face fears and guilt and overcome paranoid and obsessive thoughts, allowing energy constrictions and limitations to release. Clary Sage oil uplifts and energizes Spirit for action. It allows true joy and awe of life to manifest in all aspects of life.

Once the mental body calms, it expands quite rapidly, creating a high, euphoric feeling. Too much expansion at once may create a headache because the physical body is incapable of adjusting to the sudden increase in energy. In some people the energy of Clary Sage can induce an out of body experience, so use it with a grounding oil to maintain balance.

Using the oil for transformation

Clary Sage allows greater insights into consciousness and is a wonderful aide for clearing the mental body when used before meditation or brainstorming. Rub into the brow and temples on the head and crown chakra. This clearing allows you to clearly focus your intention. Use on the solar plexus for clearing out depression and sorrow. Inhaling the oil also revitalizes energy, so use whenever you are feeling tired for a pick-me-up. Though Clary Sage energy is stimulating for many, at the same time it is calming for the over-analytical mind.

Massaging on the lung meridian helps to reduce anxiety and anguish. Using Clary Sage oil on the triple warmer meridian helps you face the fear of the unknown by enabling the formation of new and unfamiliar thought patterns. Overcome obsessive thought patterns by massaging the oil into the large intestine meridian. Massaging into the bladder meridian along the spine reduces the tension from carrying the world's burden. Using Clary Sage oil on the kidney meridian allows people who think too much to become more focused on the moment. Stop over-thinking and ground the energy by massaging the stomach meridian with the oil. Using the oil on the gallbladder meridian releases the burden of responsibility, allowing feelings of freedom to surface. Clary Sage oil's energy helps you move through change by releasing the resistance to letting go. It is a good oil to use in mid-life crisis or for women going through the change of life. Use Clary Sage oil before a test to stimulate an energized and clear mental state.

Precautions

Avoid using during pregnancy. Do not use this oil on children or infants. Overuse of this oil can cause headaches. This oil is fairly non-irritating, to be certain check for a reaction. Use 15-30 drops in 2 ounces of a base oil.

CLOVE BUD   *Eugenia caryophyllata – Myrtaceae*
Transformations

Key: Encourages Introspection into Pain. Self-conscious behavior can comfortably transform into creative self-expression. Clove Bud releases density in the aura caused by repressed, harsh, violent, and abusive emotions and helps you feel more emotionally connected, empowering you to be true to your heart's desire and Spiritual purpose.

Growth and healing issues

Clove Bud instills an understanding of how effective it is to use power in a gentle manner. It calms the passions of inflexible and rigid people who hide their light behind defensive behavior. Clove Bud helps you reflect upon the root cause of pain, recognize how it once served you, and realize it is no longer needed. Helps in examining and overcoming the root causes of fear and anger so you may experience greater joy and spontaneity. Transforming hopelessness into faith encourages self-nourishment.

Energetic influences on the bodies and chakras

People with oral fixations benefit by using this oil. Clove oil releases stagnant energy held within the teeth, mouth, and throat chakra. Clove Bud stimulates kundalini energy to move up the spine and out the throat chakra. Anger and density held in the aura are transmuted into tranquillity.

Energetics of the oil

Clove Bud's essence has a candy-coated feeling. Its smell is medicinal with an underlying sweetness. Clove Bud oil's energy embodies power tempered with gentleness. It recalls the old adage of a velvet-covered hammer.

Clove Bud oil encourages examining the fear of expressing your self. The fear of being judged by others shuts down self-expression in many people and creates a pattern of self-consciousness.

Clove oil addresses the gnawing repressed anger that signals the presence of a denied fear. Meditating with Clove oil to discover the root cause of denied feelings can diffuse volcanic anger before it erupts. Transformation comes when you learn to feel secure expressing anger at its true cause and also from realizing that fear is what generates the anger.

Cold inner terror suppressed from early childhood experiences may surface when using Clove Bud oil. Repressed anger over time can develop into a violent streak. Energetically, Clove Bud is an excellent oil for eliminating dense repressed emotional pockets held in the aura. The energy of the oil calms the passions, allowing reflection upon the true triggers of anger. Visualizing a resolution using power of the imagination or dreams without judgment or blame is a good way to diffuse anger energy without manifesting it on the physical plane.

The energetic influence of Clove Bud oil transforms inflexible, over-thinking people by helping them recognize and overcome the inner emotional triggers that automatically engage defensive states of behavior. Clove Bud oil helps you calmly contemplate both sides of an issue.

The active warming energy of Clove Bud oil releases blockages held within the emotional body. It stimulates the Kundalini energy locked in the base of the spine to move up and out through the throat chakra. Warming the spinal energy promotes the release of tension held in the body. Clove oil also uplifts the martyr's burdensome mindset of responsibility, enabling tension held in the aura and physical body to relax. Clove Bud oil also releases the anger and rejection held within the pancreas. Meditation upon the reasons for low self-esteem releases the feelings of rejection held in the pancreas. Through meditation with Clove Bud oil you can transform feelings of hopelessness into feelings of faith. This rebuilds the connection with Spirit, allowing you to feel safe to fully feel and express emotions.

Clove Bud oil is beneficial oil to people who have given up on life. Clove oil sheds light on causes of self-defeating feelings and reasons for not taking control of your life. Use of Clove oil helps you reclaim your power and restores your appetite for life. Clove oil energy is very warming and teaches you how to receive nourishment. It teaches you to overcome the belief that life is a struggle and to want to begin caring for yourself.

Using the oil for transformation

Clove oil's nature can be overpowering; balance it by combining with a gentle calming oil. Inhale the oil and massage the liver, spleen, gallbladder, and large intestine meridians to promote the surfacing and transformation of repressed feelings. Diffuse frustrations and anger by working the oil into the gall bladder and liver meridians. Chewing Clove Buds relieves oral fixations created by and early denial of nurturing and manifested in smoking and eating disorders. Clove oil subdues parasites in the body. By giving away your power you create an opportunity for parasites to invade your body.

Use a diluted mixture of the oil on the stomach, spleen, and small intestine meridians to support self-nourishment. Inhale the oil while massaging the bladder meridian to release rigid and negative feelings. Massaging the diluted oil into the triple warmer and pericardium meridians helps overcome defensive behaviors and supports greater intimacy. Release blocked energy by massaging the conception, kidney, and stomach meridians, which stimulates the power center to open. To create a stronger desire to live, use the diluted oil on the governing and conception meridians.

Massaging Clove Bud oil on the muscle along the jaw and temple muscles brings relief from TMJ pain. Clove oil numbs the inflamed nerve tissue behind a throbbing toothache and is used traditionally to deaden dental pain. A respite from pain provides an opportunity for introspection into its emotional causes.

Precautions

Be suspicious of Clove oil's purity because it is often diluted with synthetics or less expensive constituents. This oil can irritate the skin and mucous membranes. Dilute 1-10 drops in 2 ounces of a base oil. Use only 1-5 drops in a bath. Be extra cautious when using this essential oil on children.

CYPRESS   *Cupressus sempervirens – Cupressaceae*
Transformations

Key: Maintaining Balance. Balance and freedom are realized by living in a state of acceptance. Acceptance enlightens the purpose behind all experience and promotes traveling on the path of least resistance. The importance of understanding and evaluating the effects of every choice is learned.

Growth and healing issues

Learning to maintain balance and stay centered and aligned with Spirit through raging emotional storms keeps you from being swept away and detoured from your own spiritual purpose and growth. Cultivating inner strength and determination helps you to consciously create your life. When the personality develops discriminatory abilities and the skill of Divine Right Use of Empathy, the mental body begins to disconnect from the collective consciousness.

Energetic influences on the bodies and chakras

Cypress oil helps overcome addiction to drama by energetically releasing spleen attachments, allowing greater emotional balance to be maintained. The emotional body is stimulated to respond spontaneously and joyfully. Comprehending the purpose of a karmic lesson purifies imprinted patterns in the etheric blood and rejuvenates the physical life force.

Energetics of the oil

Cypress oil energy is like standing in the eye of the hurricane. It helps you create a safe way to weather emotional storms by learning to live with the energy without owning the energy. Cypress oil enhances discernment abilities. Discernment helps you recognize where feelings originate and distinguish between your true feelings and those influenced by others. Consciously disconnecting from consensual reality helps you to live free and balanced in your own truth and reality, disconnected from other peoples' realities and thoughts. Owning your power prevents you from the distraction of other peoples' dramas, which can hinder your growth.

Energetically, Cypress oil encourages inner strength and spiritual growth and affirms the direction and purpose of your path. Cypress oil's energy supports you in making life-changing decisions and fortifies your inner strength. Cypress oil gives a consoling energy when ending all kinds of relationships. Feelings of loss are recognized as an illusion, because Spiritual doctrine proclaims nothing ever becomes lost; it only transforms.

Cypress energy helps you develop a more objective view of life. The oil enhances feelings of compassion instead of sympathy, which can feel overwhelming. Feeling overly-sympathetic can hinder your spiritual growth—in identifying with an experience you validate and accept it as your own reality. Compassion is the loving allowance of all experiences without judgment and the need to experience the situation your self. Compassion is seeing the grander cause and effect of a situation. People attract and create all of the experiences necessary for their growth. Everything has a higher purpose. People agree to play in each other's dramas to mirror their issues or bring closure to a karmic relationship. This is the wisdom of true compassion.

Energetically, Cypress disconnects spleen energy attachments. Cords and attachments are created between people through the over-empathizing, frequently when one person is attached to healing the other. This empathy energy creates karmic ties and will deplete the person attempting to do the healing work. Empathy energy is not true Source energy and carries a denser vibratory frequency.

Empathic ability does serve a purpose when in Divine Right Use. The problem is most people are unconscious empathic receivers and they take on other people's realities and ailments without realizing what they are doing. Many emotional caretakers are empathic. Making people feel better is all they know how to do, not realizing the karmic implications of their actions. When Divine Right Use is in effect, empathic abilities can provide very important diagnostic information about the energy denied or repressed into issues in the unconscious mind or emotional body. Divine Right Use employs appropriate empathizing energy and stays connected only as long as needed for interpreting information and then it fully disengages. It is up to the individual needing healing to decide how or how not to act upon the knowledge an empath imparts to them. This keeps the empathic receiver from forming karmic bonds. Empaths must make a conscious effort to train their intent to practice only Divine Right Use of empathy.

Cypress energy teaches that each course of action or thought produces a reaction, or creates a possibility that generates in time, space, and beyond. Learning to live life centered on what makes your heart sing will ultimately produce greater harmony and balance. The energy creates the reassurance of faith through certainty of knowing. It helps reestablish the ability to flow with life without the anxiety of deciding what the next step is or how it will unfold.

Women going through menopause also benefit from Cypress oil's energy. Productive energy opens up and establishes a new rhythm in their life. Cypress oil allows the energy of the etheric body to flow more efficiently into the physical. Regulation of etheric energy resolves some of the discomfort created by change.

Using the oil for transformation

Cypress oil massaged into the abdominal and colon area releases stagnant energy and beliefs held in that area. Rubbing the oil onto the forehead can reduce mental tension. Anger resolves by using the oil on the liver and gall-bladder meridians, lessening tension and increasing the energy flow through the body. Massaging Cypress oil into the gall bladder meridian (especially those points on the top of the shoulders and sides of the legs) allows tension to release.

Massaging the heart meridian with the oil helps you cope with change. Using Cypress on triple warmer meridian opens the energy for creating new behavioral patterns. Relieve the hot flashes of menopause by massaging the oil into the pericardium meridian and alleviate menstrual disorders by using the oil on the conception meridian. Massaging the oil into the large intestine meridian helps facilitate letting go.

Using Cypress on the spleen point under the left rib cage clears blockages in energy flow, and supports better assimilation of food. Massaging the oil into the spleen and spleen meridian aides in purifying the karma imprinted in the etheric blood which rejuvenates the life force of the physical body. Apply the oil to the thymus chakra above the heart and the reflex point on the hands and feet to stimulate the lymphatic system and give energy to healing karmic imprints. Rubbing the spleen area briskly in an up-and-down motion helps to seal leaking spleen energy and helps disconnect draining over-empathing energy connections with another person.

Precautions

This oil can be slightly irritating to the skin and potentially sensitizing; check for a reaction. Dilute 15-20 drops of oil in 2 ounces of base oil.

EUCALYPTUS   *Eucalyptus spp. – Myrtaceae*

Transformations

Key: Perceives Relationship Projections. The choice to consciously become Co-creators allows us to transmute karmic energy. Greater awareness about the true nature of relationships illuminates the powerful influence they have to stimulate or retard growth. Courage to transcend the collective consciousness and create a reality based on intuitive perceptions and spiritual truths is found.

Growth and healing issues

Embracing separateness allows the heart to experience a deeper state of connection. Realizing what we use as substitutes for Spiritual energy helps to release the need for dysfunctional attachments. Taking responsibility for our energy projections, and realizing the tendency they have to manipulate others, incurs true understanding of what it means to be responsible. Insight develops about our tendencies to regress into old patterns and behaviors when around family.

Energetic influences on the bodies and chakras

Eucalyptus oil works to release deep grief held in the emotional, mental, etheric, and physical bodies. The emotional and mental bodies release limitation and feelings of loss. Balance and greater assimilation occur when attuned to individual rhythms.

Energetics of the oil

Eucalyptus energy feels similar to a tropical rainforest mist. It has a cool, refreshing energy. Energetically, Eucalyptus opens the heart by aligning separation into wholeness, resulting in understanding of the importance of feeling connected to all things and generating a deeper awareness of oneness.

Eucalyptus feels refreshing and uplifting to the emotional and mental bodies. It helps release the grief held within the lungs. Intense pain and grief create a state of separation that hinder feeling other states. Mourning allows release of the loved one or furthers closure in a relationship. By not acknowledging the passing of a loved one or a relationship, the burden of grief is intensified and a feeling of loss is created. Spiritual truth proclaims that nothing can truly become lost; it only transforms from one state into another.

The energy of Eucalyptus illuminates the nature of relationships and helps us recognize dysfunctional relationship patterns. Achieving harmony and balance in relationships requires acknowledging how an attraction serves you so you may release any distorted energy attachment. Eucalyptus helps to gain an understanding of the various roles we perform to fulfill different needs in a relationship. This understanding leads to establishing healthy boundaries. Eucalyptus helps us become aware of projections and eliminate conflicts and disagreements. We no longer unconsciously manipulate someone into fulfilling our needs. Love begins with self and can only become truly filled with the spiritual Self.

Eucalyptus oil's energy heightens awareness of your connection to all life on this planet and the other realms of existence. Spiritual alignment produces greater insight into the nature of relationships and the responsibility that they require. As we become more consciously aware and responsible we take on work that has a greater impact upon life. The personality must have a clear perception of responsibility. If the personality is not ready it will not generate opportunities for experiences of great karmic influence.

Using the oil for transformation

The deep warming and penetrating abilities of Eucalyptus feel nourishing on the lungs and back of the chest. Massaging the oil into the lung meridian releases repressed feelings of grief and transforms them into joy. Making wailing sounds when inhaling the oil also promotes releasing grief.

The sinus cavities open when inhaling the oil. Closed sinus passages block the breath, cutting off the essence of life. Blocked sinuses come from unconscious issues of self-hate and subliminal death wishes. Using the oil on the governing meridian also opens blocked nasal passages. Freeing the breath lets you breathe in the essence of joy. Using the lung and sinus reflex points on the hands and feet help to open the breath. Understanding about loss comes from massaging Eucalyptus oil into the lung meridian.

Using the oil on the liver meridian helps you take responsibility for your life and destiny. Massaging the oil into the spleen and liver meridians helps to release frustration and anger created by unfulfilled needs. Applying the oil to the stomach meridian generates greater energy for self-nourishment. Massaging the oil into the small intestine meridian helps realize denied relationship needs. Release old relationship patterns by massaging the oil into the triple warmer meridian. Applying Eucalyptus to the heart and pericardium meridians helps to generate self-love. Massaging Eucalyptus onto the chest energetically expands the heart chakra.

Precautions

This oil can be slightly irritating to the skin and potentially sensitizing. Dilute 15-20 drops of oil in 2 ounces of base oil. Check for a reaction before use. Eucalyptus oil works against the effectiveness of homeopathic remedies.

FENNEL   *Foeniculum vulgare – Umbelliferae*
Transformations

Key: Realizing Substitutions for Love. Identifying what and how substitutions for love are used generates the self-love needed to overcome the lack. One learns how to properly nourish self and others with true Spiritual love.

Growth and healing issues

Fennel helps identify the root causes of self-rejection. Encourages the ability to embrace self. Feeling a lack of love in life allows substitutions for love to be used. Acknowledging the root cause of weight issues contributes to healing a poor self-image and increases self-esteem. In addition, it heals issues pertaining to victimization, dread of new ideas, and taking back one's power.

Energetic influences on the bodies and chakras

The oil stimulates the etheric thyroid by releasing feelings of insecurity and feeling out of control. It also promotes a better self-image.

Energetics of the oil

Fennel's licorice scent recalls images of an old-fashion candy store, a revealing image because Fennel conveys insightful understandings about weight issues and issues of nourishing ourselves and others.

Using Fennel in meditation recovers unconscious beliefs holding weight on the body. Often disconnection from inner strength or insecurity promotes weight gain. Holding onto hurt causes weight gain. Stagnant emotional energy solidifies into fat. Stuffing food becomes a way to avoid feelings. Releasing suppressed emotions leads to releasing blocked energy held in the lower chakras. Talking with your inner child brings clarity to some of the root-issues pertaining to weight gain. Discovering your inner child's needs provides pertinent information for achieving a greater sense of fulfillment.

The self-image a person focuses on becomes what they create. Inhaling Fennel oil during meditation gives insights into true self-image. Focusing intention and holding that energy on a projected image could change the distribution of weight. Not dealing with the root cause first will allow backsliding into the habit of stuffing food into the body.

The cultural beliefs of past lives in cultures that revered weight as a symbol of power may exist in the body memory. You might recall memories of when your were the sole provider of food for survival or fearful memories of famine or starvation in past lives. Using fennel helps recover fearful memories of not having enough. Feeling lack in life attracts behaviors of greed and gluttony. Understanding the root cause allows the weight to begin melting and food desires change.

Fennel oil also helps people with anorexia receive insights into the root cause of their behavior. Feeling unloved, unworthy or incapable of feeling love, and having a poor body image trigger anorexic behavior in some people. The root issue is a strong need to get approval and love from someone outside of Self. Breaking through this pattern of need without support can be a difficult journey. Anorexia can be fatal and it is crucial to seek professional help.

The energy of Fennel oil stimulates the thyroid. Self-esteem issues can depress the thyroid gland and create feelings of defeat, isolation, and loneliness. A person with a depressed thyroid is unable to freely express their true spiritual Self. These feelings can create the "loner" personality, a defensive behavior arising from insecurity around people. Or, another defense is a superiority complex. Fennel promotes self-acceptance and engages feelings of compassion, which results to overcome these behaviors. Meditating with Fennel oil helps relax anxieties and subdue insecurity.

Fennel's energy is the feminine equivalent of Celery oil. Using Fennel oil brings understanding about motherhood, as Celery brings insights about fatherhood. Fennel oil helps to alleviate postpartum depression. Having a new mother drink boiled fennel seeds in water helps to produce breast milk.

Fennel Seed recovers past life memories of the Isis Goddess energy in Egyptian cultures and recollection of past life memories in Mediterranean cultures.

Using the oil for transformation

A compress of diluted Fennel oil in warm or cool water placed on the eyes alleviates eye puffiness. This energetically opens the inner sight for introspection into self-esteem strength and weakness. Resistance to making life changes manifests as pain in the body. Using Fennel in a bath provides relief for physical muscular pains. Fennel oil increases stamina and endurance.

Fennel oil also helps to alleviate bloating discomforts during PMS when massaged on the stomach and lower back. Massaging oil into the bladder meridian stimulates the release of water retention.

Use of Fennel oil relieves constipation—another form of restriction and holding onto emotions. Combine Fennel oil with warm castor oil and rub it into the colon area to promote bowel movements. Using the oil on the large intestine and stomach meridians promotes letting go. Massaging on the kidney meridian unblocks energy and supports overcoming superiority and inferiority complexes by promoting self-trust. To assist developing a nourishing attitude towards self, massage the oil into the stomach, liver, and spleen meridians. Massaging the oil into the gall bladder meridian dissolves energy blockages and facilitates fat metabolism. Use on the heart and small intestine to enhance nutrient absorption and more efficient food assimilation. Oil massaged into the stomach and conception meridians clears energy obstructions and facilitates opening the power center by grounding the physical energy.

Precautions

Avoid using during pregnancy. If you have epilepsy, be careful inhaling and using externally. This oil is fairly non-irritating; check for a reaction. Use 15-30 drops in 2 ounces of a base oil. Be extra cautious when using this essential oil on children.

FIR, SIBERIAN   *Abies alba – Pinaceae*

Transformations

Key: Nurtured by the Spiritual Family. Memories of your Spiritual family awaken and their presence and love are felt. Bonding with Nature supports a better understanding for interpreting the language of life. Attuning to Nature Spirits stimulates a heightened awareness with all existence. Heightening our conscious awareness of our environment generates greater inner peace and harmony. Opening to Nature inspires taking on a co-creative role in service to all life forms. Detaching from the need to fill other people's expectations begins the process of healing the Earth family dynamics. Embracing self and life increases our self-love and promotes Spiritual growth.

Growth and healing issues

Gaining insights into childhood behaviors releases insecurity and anger. Fears that hinder Spiritual growth are addressed by introspection into the Earth family dynamics and social conditioning. Recognizing and welcoming the nurturing energy of the Spiritual family generates spiritual faith.

Energetic influences on the bodies and chakras

Acknowledging stagnant unconscious fears helps release toxins from the emotional body. A bond with Nature grounds Spiritual energy into the physical and expands the root and heart chakras. This also opens the thymus chakra permitting it to release issues that maintain our disconnection from Nature's sacredness.

Energetics of the oil

Siberian Fir's energy feels similar to being wrapped in a soft furry security blanket. The oil awakens the memory of belonging to a spiritual family and the realization that we are never alone. Energetically Fir generates Spiritual faith by releasing feelings of insecurity and loneliness. Intuition heightens with increased Spiritual faith. Remembrance of the warmth and security of the family unit brings a renewed sense of balance to the heart.

Fir is another great oil to use when we revert to childhood behaviors, as frequently occurs when we interact with our family because of the tendency to continue in roles and habits developed in past interaction. Use Fir oil to overcome the bond holding these patterns in place. Fir oil will lead to insights into the root cause and purpose of these behaviors, helping you to live life according to your truth and strengthening the bond with your Higher Self. Often we fall into old roles around our families because we believe they love who we have been and not who we are now. Accepting ourselves allows others to see our growth. Self-acceptance increases self-love and influences those around us to feel our love for them. Love attracts love and generates greater harmony and healing. Overcoming the need to play roles for other people allows them to learn responsibility for living their lives and heals family dynamics and relationships.

Fir helps in transforming feelings of self-denial into self-worth and promotes the liver to release stagnant emotional toxins. It raises awareness of fears that impede you from taking the next step in your spiritual evolution, which will allow you to feel greater joy.

Experiencing the joy of Nature increases Spiritual energy to expand into the physical. Fir opens the thymus chakra above the heart and cleanses the issues created from many lifetimes of disconnecting from the Earth's sacredness. Resolving these issues restores inner peace and harmony and establishes a greater will to live.

Fir helps a person attune to Nature Spirits. Meditating with the oil and maintaining a focused intention to experience Nature Spirits initiates communication with the Elves, Gnomes, and Pan energy. An understanding of the messages coming from trees, flowers, birds, and animals grows daily and expands the heart chakra. A feeling of bliss and love grows strong in a person's entire being and creates a deep bond of respect for the essence of Mother Nature. Fir promotes a desire to participate in more outdoor activities, which will stimulate more environmental consciousness. Co-creation is humanity's responsibility and Fir helps you understand your role in the service to Nature. This Divine Right Order will enable the restoration of harmony and love on the planet.

Using the oil for transformation

Siberian Fir massaged on the liver meridian releases anger. Rubbing into the heels opens and grounds the Earth connection. Using Fir oil on the stomach meridian helps to bring balance to the Earth element within you. Align the energy for living in the present and heighten the ability to communicate with Nature by using Fir oil on the kidney meridian

Massaging Fir into the heart and pericardium meridians promotes a feeling of nourishment and establishing greater intimacy in relationships.

Rub into the thymus while gently tapping the area to stimulate the immune system. This also generates greater memory of multidimensionality and parallel lives simultaneously existing on the Earth plane. Siberian Fir encourages Self-discovery of true magnificence. Fir on the triple warmer meridian energy warms feelings generated by social and family ties. Opening this energy also stimulates the desire for developing new relationship patterns.

Precautions

Fir oil can be slightly irritating to the skin and potentially sensitizing; check for a reaction. Dilute 15-20 drops of oil in 2 ounces of base oil.

FRANKINCENSE   *Bosellia carteri – Burseraceae*
Transformations

Key: Awakens Spiritual Purpose. Soul memories can instill serenity. Spiritual purpose awakens and aligns with the personality, enhancing the bond with Soul. This connection produces spiritual integrity and responsibility, leading to increased Spiritual growth towards mastery. The boundaries of time and space are transcended by focusing intention on experiencing other realms.

Growth and healing issues

Ancient memories awaken arousing wisdom and parting the veils held over the consciousness. Doors open to other realms of consciousness. Taking responsibility for actions establishes integrity and a conscious choice of intention. Acknowledgment of denied emotions generates Spiritual growth. The personality's impatience is resolved by learning lessons that end the repetition of painful and frustrating experiences. The bondage of denial is released with honest introspection to comprehend the purpose of a lesson or experience.

Energetic influences on the bodies and chakras

The life force in the physical body is amplified by increased oxygenation that nurtures and rejuvenates the physical organs. The crown, third eye, and heart chakras expand as new realities are perceived. The light body enlarges by experiencing new realities and dimensions.

Energetics of the oil

Frankincense's name and scent awaken ancient memories. Energetically it arouses remembrance of wisdom, parting the veil held over the consciousness. Frankincense oil reveals memories of Soul experiences.

Meditation with Frankincense oil awakens Spiritual purpose in a person. Frankincense's energy in religious ceremonies through the ages has helped people to feel closer to God's mercy. It was widely believed that burning Frankincense raised prayers to heaven. Using the oil guides and reconnects person into their God essence, known as the I Am presence.

Energetically Frankincense helps a person develop the integrity to take responsibility for the consequences of their actions. Not learning the lesson of an experience hinders Spiritual growth and may cause a painful, frustrating repetition of events.

The Magi gave the gift of Frankincense to the baby Jesus. Traditionally Frankincense eases childbirth, the instrumental process of manifesting life from one dimension to another. The oil's aroma encourages exploring different dimensions and realities. Frankincense energy carries a person across the barriers of time and space. The Soul does not operate in the constraints of time and space. From the Soul's point of view all incarnations occur simultaneously and only the personality dies with the body. Comprehending the Soul's immortality generates patience and the realization that impatience is a personality characteristic.

The Frankincense tree grows in the desert. The starkness of the desert landscape helps people to feel the serenity of their Soul. Energetically, the oil recalls memories of many ancient cultures of the Middle East, especially those of the collective consciousness of Arabia and the wandering Bedouin tribes, and memories in the era of Solomon.

Using the oil for transformation

Inhaling Frankincense oil combined with breath exercises helps still the conscious mind for connecting with the God essence. To connect a person with their path of spiritual pursuit use the oil on the heart and pericardium meridians. Using the oil on the heart, lung, triple warmer, and large intestine meridians allows easier transitions of life. Use the oil on the small intestine meridian to increase vitality in the body and mind. Massaging oil on the liver meridian integrates the whole self. Frankincense oil used on the spleen meridian energizes and balances the body's energy.

Working with this oil on the liver and gall bladder meridians can help one develop integrity and take responsibility for feelings and actions. Massaging Frankincense into the kidney helps to ground the body into the moment while strengthening spiritual purpose. The oil massaged into the heart and lung meridians promotes greater oxygenation into the body's organs. Inhale Frankincense oil to oxygenate the breath and revitalize all the organs. Use the oil to free energy constrictions in the conception and governing meridians to gently release unconscious fear and terror of being in the physical. Massaging Frankincense into the triple warmer meridian connects the hypothalamus with the pituitary gland and heightens the third eye intuitive perceptions.

Precautions

Frankincense oil is fairly non-irritating, to be certain check for a reaction. Use 15-30 drops in 2 ounces of a base oil.

GERANIUM (ROSE)   *Pelargonium graveolens – Geraniaceae*

Transformations

Key: Eases Heartache. Nurturing and soothing the forsaken parts of self stimulates a sense of safety, encouraging the desire to emotionally relate with others. Embracing feelings of embarrassment that contribute to low self-esteem leads to greater self-acceptance. Increasing self-acceptance generates a greater sense of resourcefulness and self fulfillment. Learning to love oneself allows Soul fragments to reunite with the God essence of Self, resolving internal conflict.

Growth and healing issues

Initiates an energetic confrontation of the issues that cause conflict, heartache, and abandonment, which allows the fragmented Self to become integrated into the Higher Self's wholeness. Feelings from a broken heart, such as abandonment and isolation, are eased by validating and embracing those parts. Embracing Divine Grace transforms deep feelings of shame and unworthiness into love and acceptance.

Energetic influences on the bodies and chakras

Heart energy expands by experiencing the freedom of joyous love. The personality integrates with the Soul essence. Expanding and opening the thymus chakra recalls memories of injustices experienced in past lifetimes. Judgment of those actions suppresses the thymus and immune system. Rips and holes in the emotional body caused by discordant emotions begin to heal by strengthening the bond with Soul energy.

Energetics of the oil

Rose Geranium energy invokes the joy of watching a butterfly on a hot summer day. The energy summons the emotional feelings of freedom produced from a joyful heart. The oil's association with the planet Venus revitalizes the essence of love into a person's life.

Energetically it stimulates the energy of Divine Grace to ease the influence that feelings of shame and humiliation produce. Surrendering into the acceptance of those feelings develops the understanding that all experiences are part of the journey. Memories of all lifetimes are embedded into the cellular-memory of the thymus chakra. This is a dormant chakra that awakens when multi-dimensional perceptions include access to Akashic records. When this chakra is activated past life memories surface. Judging memories from any lifetime's action depresses the immune system and contributes to feelings of unworthiness. The energetics of Geranium oil expand the thymus chakra letting injustices heal. Looking at the experience as a lesson on the journey releases the bondage and karma created by holding blame against those involved. An expanded thymus chakra also enhances self-acceptance and awakens resourcefulness.

Geranium oil has a very gentle nurturing energy that works on the Soul level. It energetically heals rips and holes in the emotional body created by strong discordant emotions. The energy of Rose Geranium soothes heartache and overcomes feelings of abandonment and rejection by validating and nurturing the parts of Self that feel forsaken. Integrating these forsaken parts into the Soul's essence of wholeness diminishes internal conflict and allows greater self-love. This manifests the I Am presence.

Using the oil for transformation

Rose Geranium feels wonderfully nurturing when used on the heart and breasts. Apply the oil to the sides of the rib cage and under the breast to stimulate greater self-acceptance. Using the oil on the kidney meridian generates greater self-trust. Massaging the oil into the pineal gland reflex point on the hands and feet stimulates cellular regeneration. Use the oil while stimulating the pineal point between the eyebrows and above the bridge of the nose.

Precautions

Be suspicious of Geranium oil's purity because it is often diluted with synthetics or less expensive constituents. This oil is fairly non-irritating; check for a reaction. Use 15-30 drops in 2 ounces of a base oil.

GINGER   *Zingiber officinalis – Zingiberaceae*
Transformations

Key: Realizes the Sacred Self. Encouraging the hidden and vulnerable parts of the personality towards the light promotes recognition of the most sacred parts of self. Reducing resistance to change establishes harmony and balance. Strengthening and grounding Spiritual energy awakens memories of past life talents and lets them become resources in the present.

Growth and healing issues

Opening the inner eye allows perception of the shadow self. This perception transforms insecurities, fears, and denied feelings of grief and loss. Acknowledging denied feelings of hurt and ridicule allows realization of how these feelings manifest as reactions. Befriending the inner child stimulates emotional healing.

Energetic influences on the bodies and chakras

Ginger produces etheric enzymes allowing new realities to be easily digested and assimilated. Recognizing the sacred parts of Self opens and expands the crown chakra. More light absorbs into the physical body when crown energy aligns with all the chakras. Integrating the first and second chakras with the heart energy transforms suppressed sexual energy into creative or healing energy. The etheric first chakra expands, generating a more stable and grounded state.

Energetics of the oil

Ginger grows in diverse shapes, colors, and forms. The tropical flowers have a delightful, enchanting fragrance. The spice comes from the tubular root and symbolically correlates to the unconscious mind. Ginger promotes feelings of sacredness. Energetically, it helps recognize the deeply sacred part of Self called the Higher Self or Spirit.

Ginger guides the hidden vulnerable parts of the personality towards the light. These are the parts of the self that retain the memories of being hurt or ridiculed. Repressed fears, grief, and guilt develop the shadow self's density. Ginger heals the shadow part of the personality by heightening third eye energy and stimulating the light to transform the shadow self. This alignment of energy encourages the fragile parts of self to bloom. Meditating with Ginger oil transforms the shadow self's fears and insecurities.

Ginger oil's energy uncovers denied or unconscious feelings of grief stemming from a broken heart or a loss of innocence. Ginger eases the intense feelings of transitional pubescent and teenager states and subdues the energy of childish temper tantrums. Ginger oil combined with inner child therapies promotes rapid emotional healing. Acknowledging the inner child and introducing it to an environment of love and protection empowers the whole Self to feel safe and secure.

Ginger releases grief held in the lungs and the emotional body. Its warming energy clears mucus and stimulates the healing of coughs and colds. The dense and cloudy nature of mucus blocks the light within. Expelling mucus allows more light to radiate outward. Inhaling Ginger oil stimulates etheric digestive enzymes and promotes easier assimilation of new energies.

The aphrodisiac nature of Ginger opens the first chakra and unleashes suppressed sexual energy. Elevating sexual energy vibrations and integrating it with the heart and crown chakras transforms it into healing energy or creativity. Ginger opens the crown chakra and aligns and infuses all the chakras with Spiritual energy.

The energy of Ginger awakens memories of lifetimes spent in Polynesian, Tahitian, and Lemurian cultures. Ginger's rich history includes a tradition of use in ritual magic. It supports recollection of great spiritual strengths and grounds that ancient knowledge in the present. Using Ginger oil can access abilities developed in other lives as resources for the present life.

Using the oil for transformation

Ginger promotes release of toxins through sweating and has a diuretic effect on the physical body. Massage into areas like the ankles and fingers where water is often retained. Use on the kidney and bladder meridians to release stagnant water from the body, which also stimulates releasing repressed emotions. With gentle pressure manipulate the bladder and kidney reflex points on the hands and feet to free constricted energy. Clear mucus and open up the lung energy by using Ginger oil on the lung and colon meridians. This also induces deeper breathing nourishing all the physical organs. Using Ginger oil on the lung, stomach, and large intestine meridians eases fears asthmatics may have about relating to others.

Massaging the body with the oil stimulates the circulation and increases etheric energy to replenish the physical. Ginger's energy engages the immune system on the etheric level and increases vitality. Massaging Ginger oil on cold parts of the body creates a warming sensation and moves blocked emotional energy.

Precautions

Ginger oil can irritate the skin and mucous membranes. Dilute 1-10 drops in 2 ounces of a base oil before applying to the skin. Use only 1-5 drops in a bath.

GRAPEFRUIT   *Citrus x paradisi – Rutaceae*

Transformations

Key: Calms Mental Chatter. Calming mind chatter helps to clearly hear the Inner Source's directives and heightens clairaudience. Determining the origin of beliefs helps release their karmic imprint. Developing discernment skills helps make choices, as opposed to reactions.

Growth and healing issues

Becoming more conscious of your mental chatter leads to discovering how powerful and overwhelming an influence it is on your self-esteem and how it contributes to fragmenting the personality, maintaining a state of confusion. Lifting depression eases resistance to change.

Energetic influences on the bodies and chakras

Clearing the density in the aura and mental body created by thought forms allows you to clearly hear inner source, enabling you to become more directed by Soul purpose. Calming the mental body expands the heart and third eye chakras, resulting in a harmonious assimilation of new energies influential in creating new realities.

Energetics of the oil

Grapefruit has a tangy refreshing sensation that rejuvenates the core of a person's being. Energetically it dissipates thought forms held in the aura, making this oil a powerful mental body cleanser.

Constant mind chatter causes overwhelmed and confused states of mind. Mind chatter is a like a tape recording of negative programming: voices, pictures, or feelings that perpetuate to reinforce old behaviors and thoughts and resist any type of change. These tapes are often detrimental to self-esteem and hinder the ability to be decisive. Overcoming mind chatter is possible with constant attention to what you are saying to yourself. Conscious awareness of these messages will help identify their source and whether they are pertinent to the current situation. The mind needs conscious reprogramming to establish and maintain a new consciousness. To stop the detrimental messages whenever an old tape begins to play, push your mental delete button. Reaffirming to your self that these thoughts are old and inappropriate responses helps to stop the program loop. Use Grapefruit oil in meditation and validate your new reality by stating "I love and embrace that old thought but it no longer serves me." Over time the mind stops playing those old programs and lets you make choices as opposed to simply reacting.

Calming mind chatter lets you clearly hear Inner Source, promoting a clearer direction actualized by spiritual purpose and expands the heart chakra, releasing constricted energy created by judging thoughts. The third eye chakra also expands, heightening intuitive perception for clarity.

Energetically Grapefruit removes karmic imprints from the etheric blood. The cleansing energy lifts any depressive thought patterns maintaining unnecessary karmic bonds. Frequently these thoughts spring from a past life reality bleeding into the present reality. These imprinted thought patterns may also develop from family and social conditioning, crystallized over time. Overcoming these thought patterns empowers you to establish your unique present reality. This also aids development of spiritual focus and an understanding of how to participate in service to enlighten humanity. Grounding these new energies into the physical lets you enact them. The energy of Grapefruit oil also helps assimilate the astrological energies of a Mercury retrograde. The mind becomes calmer, lessening the confusion the retrograde energies create.

Grapefruit oil is both anti-fungal and anti-parasitic. On a spiritual level, it heals the issues allowing fungus and parasites to invade the body. Fungal conditions come from accepting other peoples' beliefs to control your life, parasitic conditions ripen giving your power over to others. Grapefruit energy restores and establishes responsibility for your power, helping to develop your unique abilities and clarify your spiritual purpose.

Using the oil for transformation

Massaging Grapefruit oil into the temples and forehead calms the mental body. Using Grapefruit oil enhances clairaudience. Rubbing the oil behind the ears and on the kidney meridian opens the etheric ear. Anointing the crown and third eye chakras enhances the ability to perceive Source. Feeling physical tightness in neck and shoulder areas comes from mental stress; massaging the oil on the area helps lesson the tension. Massaging along the triple warmer meridian also helps to alleviate shoulder pain and stiffness. Applying on the stomach meridian calms the mental stress of thinking too much. Massaging on the spleen meridian releases karmic imprints, worry, and anxiety.

Precautions

This oil can be slightly irritating to the skin and potentially sensitizing. Check for a reaction. Dilute 15-20 drops of oil in 2 ounces of base oil.

HELICHRYSUM (EVERLASTING, IMMORTELLE)

Helichrysum angustifolium—Asteraceae

Transformations

Key: Conscious Empowerment and Initiation. Stimulates comprehension of the Soul's immortality that overcomes the personality's lack of patience. Supports greater Spiritual integration within the physical, which promotes the human experience to progress through the seven levels of consciousness. The progression of evolution and the basic foundations needed to achieve each level become understood. Greater balance becomes experienced as you move closer to your true Spiritual nature enhancing your ability to see all sides of an experience.

Growth and healing issues

Addresses the frustration of separation from Spirit. Provides assistance for transcending into the consciousness of the Initiated. Helps to understand the spiraling forces that direct energy through the seven levels of consciousness — Tribal, Mass, Individual, Aspirant, Disciple, Initiate, and Master. Illuminates the inherent challenges that each level of consciousness incurs.

Energetic influences on the bodies and chakras

Aids in releasing the energy distortions caused by the experience of each level of consciousness. Helps to integrate the energy by remembering the lessons that each level of consciousness has taught you on the journey of self-discovery.

Energetics of the oil

The scent of Helichrysum oil embodies the sweetness of Spirit. Energetically it empowers the journey of self-discovery. The oil's energy awakens remembrance of the Soul's long journey, inspiring the personality to integrate with Spirit. This oil promotes living life with greater conscious awareness by overcoming the frustration of separation from Spirit.

Energetically, Helichrysum oil accesses esoteric knowledge buried in the unconscious. This knowledge is revealed in teachings received through dreams, meditation, or contact with other dimensional Beings. It opens thinking and acting on an Initiate level of consciousness. An Initiate is not bound to the limitation of mass consciousness and strives to Co-Create with all life forms. Living life joyously with the ability to laugh at yourself maintains this consciousness.

Helichrysum oil achieves greater Spiritual integration within the physical and promotes rapid progress through the seven levels of consciousness. Progressing through the levels of consciousness creates a spiraling energy pattern of Spiritual evolution. Belief in your Self is necessary to find the courage to overcome the limitations of consensual reality. Use Helichrysum to help integrate the solar plexus with the heart chakra, which Will to be directed by Spiritual intention. Helichrysum energy helps to overcome feelings of unworthiness by anchoring the sweetness of Spirit.

As we expand up the spiral of consciousness, each level stimulates an initiation. Each initiation is a new experience for the journey. As more people move through these initiations it increases the radiance of higher frequencies of vibration, the experience of Love or Light. As evolution continues and more light is anchored the limitations of the physical world as we know it will be transcended, actualizing a greater embodiment of the Light.

Using the oil for transformation

Meditation with Helichrysum oil helps you integrate and remember the lessons that each level of consciousness contains, promoting easier passage through the initiations. Pain arises from holding onto beliefs that no longer serve you and blocks your passage into the higher initiations. Energetically, Helichrysum oil instills the courage to powerfully manifest with Spiritual intention. Use Helichrysum oil when going through any initiation or rite. Meditating with the oil enlightens the true meaning of each initiation. Helichrysum energy helps to lift the veils held over consciousness, promoting spiritual evolution. You feel greater balance in life when you move closer to your true Spiritual nature and gain the ability to see the truth of experience.

Precautions

This oil can be slightly irritating to the skin and potentially sensitizing. Check for a reaction. Dilute 15-20 drops of oil in 2 ounces of base oil.

HYSSOP   *Hyssopus officinalis – Labiatae*
Transformations

Key: Perception of the Spiritual Self. Expanding and heightening perception supports inner strength and the courage needed to follow the heart's desires. Fortifying Spiritual purpose lights the path of self-discovery. Understanding Divine Right Timing is achieved by acknowledging the perfection of life. Learning a lesson produces Spiritual growth and generates greater self-acceptance.

Growth and healing issues

Purging old beliefs that do not serve Spiritual growth calms the internal struggle of conflicting realities. The burdens of guilt and duty are felt as a limitation, which intensifies fears and constricts the nervous system. Increasing self-acceptance overcomes unworthiness and generates compassion.

Energetic influences on the bodies and chakras

The emotional, mental, physical, and etheric bodies begin to release the density of fear. Confusion resolves by clearing the density around the aura caused by mental chatter. The energy purifies and sanctifies spaces for rituals. When the personality desires to integrate with the Higher Self more Spirit manifests.

Energetics of the oil

The scent of Hyssop directly stimulates third eye energy. It enables a rapid expansion of perceptive abilities and the acknowledgment that Spirit is the directing force. Energetically Hyssop fortifies your resolve to walk your path. It supports the courage needed to follow your heart's desire and the endurance needed for Self-discovery. Hyssop opens the energy to manifest the Higher Self through the personality.

Hyssop is associated with the energy of the winter solstice. Use Hyssop during the winter because that is Nature's period of introspection. Rebirth comes by sweeping out the old, creating a space for receiving new energy. Hyssop helps to purge realities that are no longer useful to the self, calming the internal stress caused by conflicting realities. Energetically, Hyssop works to clear out the resonance of realities long outgrown. It clears the mental body and aura of debris that contribute to constant mind chatter and confusion. Releasing these old thought patterns heightens the ability to focus intention more intensely.

Hyssop oil initiates Divine self-acceptance and attracts the gaiety and mirth that are lost when carrying the burdens of guilt and duty. Hyssop expands lung energy by releasing guilt. It soothes bronchial conditions by increasing the capacity to breathe more deeply. Energetically Hyssop oil allows discovery of intense fears held in the unconscious mind by releasing stress held in the nervous system and allowing the realization of how fears have constricted nerves over time. Hyssop teaches you to be gentler with Self and not be so stern and rigid. It lessens the drive behind convictions and permits the energy to ease into relaxation. This is a good oil for "Type A" personalities, as it leads them to understanding they are the cause of their own internal pressure. When they comprehend the root of their need to be perfect, self-acceptance and compassionate tolerance are stimulated. Hyssop helps you comprehend that errors are part of learning the process and there are no mistakes. Errors are recognized as true blessings in the perfection of Divine Right Timing.

Hyssop oil was traditionally used to purify sacred spaces. Use Hyssop oil for initiation ceremonies or occasions marking important milestones in life. It creates a feeling of reverence for the occasion. Hyssop purifies the etheric, emotional, physical, and mental bodies. By purifying all aspects of the Self, the energy of the subtle bodies is aligned and flows harmoniously into the physical body. Hyssop releases the burden of sins and the imagined guilt they produce lifting the heavy hindrance of unworthiness.

Hyssop recalls memories of Pagan and Essene lifetimes. Pagans used Hyssop to purify their temples, as did the Catholic Church. Holy Water was sprinkled with sprigs of Hyssop, especially onto clean feet. The ritual of washing feet symbolizes the purification that the Holy Spirit manifests into a person's life. Hyssop helps prepare for rituals and ceremonies requiring a meditative state for connecting with the Higher Self, especially purifying baths.

Using the oil for transformation

Use Hyssop for any type of purification, especially for rooms that contain charged emotion or depression. Add the oil to water and spray the mixture in the room to uplift and transmute the dense thought forms vibrating in the space.

Rubbing Hyssop oil on the shoulder helps reduce the tension from carrying emotional burdens. Using the oil on the small intestine meridian will increase energy vitality. Hyssop oil used on the lung and large intestine meridians releases mucus congestion in the lungs and bronchial tubes and purges grief held within the subtle body's energy. Using Hyssop on the lung reflex points of the hands and feet helps break up congestion produced by inwardly grieving. Massaging with deep pressure into the colon reflex points of the hands and feet helps release stagnated energy from the colon and purges toxins from the physical body. Energizing the liver, spleen, and large intestine meridians by massaging the oil into them releases physical toxins.

Precautions

Do not use Hyssop on pregnant women because it could cause a miscarriage. Do not use on children or infants. If you have epilepsy, be careful inhaling and using externally. If high blood pressure is present, use cautiously in baths and highly diluted as a massage oil, but do not inhale.

JUNIPER   *Juniperus communis – Cupressaceae*

Transformations

Key: Strengthens Spiritual Will. Developing greater patience generates the ability to feel comfortable in the stillness of Spirit. Renewing the connection with your Soul group creates an alignment with Source, guiding life by Source instead of by the personality's whims.

Growth and healing issues

Energetically aids feeling the security and protection that your Soul group provides, thus inspiring greater reverence for all of life's experiences. Releases unconscious feelings of anger, frustration, annoyance, and anxiety and increases unconditional love.

Energetic influences on the bodies and chakras

Aligning the Spiritual will with the personality channels more light from the etheric body into the physical body. This expansion stimulates increased consciousness. The heart chakra begins to align with Source.

Energetics of the oil

Juniper inspires the vision of a Mexican God's eye. The eye is a religious relic that symbolically asks God to lovingly watch over someone. Visualizing the symbol while using the oil reinforces feelings of security.

Juniper oil attunes you to the subtle energies that are saturating your aura. These energies may originate from your Soul group or other Energies of Light assisting you on the path of self-discovery. Acknowledging the Unseen Realm helps overcome the fear and loneliness that losing faith produces. It supports a greater understanding of Source, inspiring sacred feelings of reverence.

Juniper energetically increases the crystalline light structure of the etheric body, creating an expansion of consciousness. With this expansion, more light assimilates into the physical body, bringing deeper feelings of unconditional love. Many people have allergies to the juniper tree, which is symptomatic of hardening themselves against feeling love. Juniper oil cleanses and purifies the emotional body of stagnant thought patterns of anger, frustration, annoyance, and uncertainty by kindling the fire essence in your being. This essence fortifies and purifies the Spiritual Will. Juniper was burned for purification in ancient Tibetan rituals.

Using Juniper oil recalls memories of Pagan lifetimes. Its energy attracts Fairies and Elves into your life. Legends proclaim that Juniper trees guarded the entrance to the Other Worlds.

Using the oil for transformation

Massaging Juniper oil into the small and large intestine meridians, spleen meridian, and kidney meridian helps release blocked energy held in the physical body. Use on the bladder and governing meridians for help overcoming feelings of terror. Juniper oil massaged into the liver meridian lifts feelings of boredom, stubbornness, and anger. Burning Juniper oil in an aromatherapy lamp or diffuser helps to purify a room. To stimulate energy, hold any tender meridian points and visualize Source energy running through them.

Precautions

Avoid using during pregnancy. Do not use this oil on children or infants. Diabetics should be cautious of this oil. Juniper is often diluted with turpentine. Juniper oil can be slightly irritating to the skin and potentially sensitizing; check for a reaction. Dilute 15-20 drops of oil in 2 ounces of base oil. Juniper oil may be problematic for people who suffer with allergies and asthma.

LAUREL LEAF, BAY LAUREL   *Laurus nobilis – Lauraceae*

Transformations

Key: Heightens Perception Abilities. Greater self-trust heightens intuitive abilities, especially clairaudience and clairvoyance. The mind better understands abstract thought and messages, which stimulates creativity. Shifting your focus to different realities cultivates perception of infinite possibilities.

Growth and healing issues

Learning the right use of power increases discernment abilities. Learning to discern energy, and trusting the process of acquiring this information, heightens the ability to intuitively know. Learning to trust and honor Self reclaims personal power and generates greater inner peace.

Energetic influences on the bodies and chakras

Integrating the emotional and mental bodies produces a greater reception and trust of intuitive information. Relaxing the mental body's control over the thought process brings inner peace. Balancing and opening the sacral chakra and aligning its energy with the throat chakra better articulates creative thought.

Energetics of the oil

Laurel leaves braided into a crowning wreath were given to the "poet laureate" and to victorious athletes in the ancient Olympics. The essence of Laurel oil supports the ability to honor your self.

Laurel was also associated with prophecy and divination. Laurel oil stimulates intuitive abilities of clairaudience and clairvoyance. The energetics of Laurel awaken discernment, which builds trust in the unconscious aspects of self. Energetically Laurel works to integrate the emotional body with the mental body. The mental body's need for logical proof tends to invalidate or block intuitions received from the emotional body. Laurel oil harmonizes the mental body to exist with the emotional intuitive body. In addition, Laurel oil helps connect with stronger feelings of inner peace.

Laurel oil also helps overcome the fear of claiming personal power. This fear could be rooted in a past life experience of abusing power or current social conditioning against handling power. Developing intuition and discernment helps you reclaim power.

Laurel oil awakens the desire for artistic endeavors. The oil opens the throat chakra's expression, enhancing creativity, and opens and balances the sacral chakra, amplifying fertility of thought. The part of the etheric brain controlling creativity begins to vibrate at a higher frequency. Meditation with Laurel oil inspires the creativity to achieve life's needs and desires.

Laurel Leaf awakens memories of ancient Greek and Roman lifetimes, as well as lives in the Renaissance.

Using the oil for transformation

A bath with Laurel oil relieves arthritic symptoms, dissolving resistance to change held in the emotional and mental bodies. Meditation with Laurel helps overcome limitations in thought and unleash creativity. Massaging the small intestine meridian with the oil will also help open up creativity. Using the oil on the heart and lung meridians helps you honor your self. Spray Laurel oil in the room to stimulate the environmental energy to vibrate at the Higher Mind's frequency when trying to manifest abstract thought.

Precautions

This oil can be slightly irritating to the skin and potentially sensitizing; check for a reaction. Dilute 15-20 drops of oil in 2 ounces of base oil.

LAVENDER   *Lavandula angustifolia – Labiatae*
Transformations

Key: Soothes Grief and Promotes Peace. Trance channeling abilities heighten, bringing intuitive information from new sources. Easing tension allows creating new perceptions. The Unseen Realm feels closer and contact is realized.

Growth and healing issues

Learning to relax produces greater inner peace and harmony. Stress is calmed by soothing the passions that create turmoil and by easing the grief of heartache. Diminishing the emotional intensity of memories allows a feeling of security. Clearer communication between the mind and body restores inner trust.

Energetic influences on the bodies and chakras

Lavender energy lovingly embraces all the bodies with peace and flows through the subtle bodies, channeling greater aspects of Self into reality. The heart and crown chakras simultaneously open, expand, and align to anchor calmness and peace. Releasing tension and stress allows the dreaming body to freely explore the labyrinths of the astral planes.

Energetics of the oil

Lavender feels similar to a gentle nourishing spring rain. Energetically Lavender oil feels very wise, like an elder, or like a loving embrace of deep peace. When calmness prevails, healing begins. Use of Lavender heals the passions that create much of the turmoil and grief in life.

The energy of Lavender oil has a soothing gentleness that eases the heart and inspires calm and new perspectives. Tension ebbs away and greater spiritual energy courses through all the subtle bodies, enabling greater aspects of Self to manifest into reality. Lavender promotes trance channeling. Using this oil with a focused intention initiates the simultaneous opening of the crown chakra and the heart chakra, which generates feelings of calmness and peace. Lavender teaches lessons of patience within the framework of eternity.

Lavender can be a soothing balm to memories. Its inspires feelings of security, much like having a guardian presence around. Meditating with Lavender oil helps people attune with their guardian Angels. Using at night induces sweet dreams and leads the dreaming body through the labyrinths of the astral plane. It helps a dreamer remember the teachings of dream states. Lavender establishes channels of communication between the conscious and unconscious minds, helping to build trust in Self.

Using the oil for transformation

Use Lavender on the crown chakra on the top of the head to release the built-up physical pressure and promote relaxation. Using the oil on the heart chakra allows feelings of grace. Lavender massaged on the temples and forehead helps bring calm into a person's life. Rubbing Lavender on the body while applying pressure on the intersection of the bridge of the nose and brow helps alleviate depression. When a person is in a state of hysteria, anoint and hold the depression on the edge of the wrist bones. Gentle Lavender soothes the thymus gland. Use on the lung meridian to release grief and nourish the emotions.

Precautions

This oil is fairly non-irritating; to be certain check for a reaction. Use 15-30 drops in 2 ounces of a base oil. Overuse of Lavender oil may cause headaches.

LEMON   *Citrus limon – Rutaceae*

Transformations

Key: Increases Inner Joy and Optimism. The throat chakra clears, allowing proficient self-expression. The mind sharpens, grasping abstract thought that brings Spirit into action.

Growth and healing issues

Generating inner joy transforms pessimism into optimism. Greater wisdom is realized by learning to focus untrained and scattered mental energy. Wisdom inspires a sense of hope that transforms cynicism and confusion.

Energetic influences on the bodies and chakras

Alcohol addiction is released from the cellular memory. Lemon is a cleansing balm to all bodies and lifts depressed moods.

Energetics of the oil

Lemon energy is a bright yellow ball of sunshine. Lemon oil creates feelings of nuturing warmth that inspire a lasting feeling of great inner joy. Lemon brightens a soured disposition and can make pessimistic people more optimistic. Cynical people expect the worst, often because their life challenges have not worked out the way they wanted. Heartburn often manifests from cynical feelings lodged in the liver and gallbladder. Energetically Lemon inspires optimism, encouragement, and a sense of hope, transforming cynicism held in the consciousness.

Lemon energy is a paradox because it energizes and calms simultaneously. Lemon focuses frantic and scattered energy, creating a feeling of deep nourishment. Lemon clears the mental body of confusion and fills with golden Spiritual consciousness. Lemon enhances the ability to comprehend abstract thought and manifest it into action. Its energy promotes mental agility and is beneficial to people who must make quick decisions.

Lemon opens and clears the throat chakra. The blue color of the throat chakra combined with the yellow color of Lemon creates turquoise, a higher-frequency energy that effectively commands self-expression.

Lemon oil's cleansing properties release toxins in the liver. Lemon oil may be used to cleanse the cellular memory of alcoholics and children of alcoholics and can transform the unconscious death wishes of this addiction. As with all potentially addictive substances there is a Divine Right use that transforms adverse reactions. Focusing on using a substance with proper intent instead of judging a behavior as repulsive and bad, leads to overcoming addition. Realizing a part of the self is generating the addictive behavior and loving that part of self helps overcome its need to continue the habit.

Lemon's essence helps to clean the etheric layer of the Aura. The Aura contains pranic threads of energy that surround the physical body. These energy threads of light are created by the continual transference of energy through the bodies. Confused and scattered thoughts tangle the threads. Using Lemon oil untangles the pranic threads, enabling more focus.

Using the oil for transformation

Use Lemon on the liver and gallbladder meridians to remove obstructions in energy and increase the life force. Gently massage Lemon oil on the gall-bladder points of the forehead and the liver points to release headache pressure. Massaging the oil on the liver meridian and into the womb relieves PMS symptoms. Lemon is a great liver cleanser and will help alcoholics to detoxify and release their cravings.

Lemon clears the air of an emotionally charged space. The smell of Lemon shifts the mood of an environment. Lemon oil can be used to cheer up sick people in a hospital. Drinking hot water with Lemon and honey soothes stress in the vocal cords—a remedy for singers and performers that also helps them express their talents.

Precautions

This oil can be slightly irritating to the skin and potentially sensitizing; keep exposure to sunlight at a minimum. Dilute 15-20 drops of oil in 2 ounces of base oil. The candy-like smell will attract children; keep it away from them. Do not use this oil on children or infants.

LEMON GRASS   *Cymbopogon citrates and flexes – Gardenia*
Transformations

Key: Spirit Lights the Conscious Mind. Optimism generates the courage to overcome any situation. A pessimistic outlook dissipates, restoring flexibility for dealing with challenging experiences. Clearing and calming the mind stimulates attitudes that lead to Spiritual growth.

Growth and healing issues

The nervous system is calmed while the mind is simultaneously stimulated. Clearing the conscious mind stimulates left brain functions and encourages a more concise actualization of self. Stressful anxieties about the future dissolve into patience and confidence.

Energetic influences on the bodies and chakras

The crown chakra expands and spiritualizes the thought process. Lemon Grass is an energetic tonic to the etheric body and shields the aura from electromagnetic bombardment.

Energetics of the oil

Lemon Grass's scent has an uplifting clean sensation that penetrates deep into the body. To the mind, the energy feels like a breath of spring air, brushing out cobwebs so sunshine beams into the conscious mind.

The energetics of Lemon Grass oil soften rigid mental attitudes, changing a pessimistic outlook to one of optimism. It anchors the ability to be more flexible in thought, promoting a hopeful and receptive disposition. Resistance to change restricts spiritual progress. Often change is felt as a loss. Shifting this attitude into one of joy and adventure allows a dramatic leap in spiritual growth. Lemon Grass stimulates the left brain, tempering concrete logical thoughts with Spirituality by energetically opening the crown chakra and enabling the brain to expand and open new pathways. Increasing spiritual energy in the left brain helps manifest ideas into form. This energy is instrumental for actualizing Self in a concise and directed manner.

Lemon Grass sedates the nervous system while stimulating the mind. It combats stress by cleaning and purifying the etheric body, which helps dissipate the dense energy of stress. Often stress is generated by living in the rat race and the pressures of life in today's society. Lemon Grass helps overcome depression rooted in trying to live up to social standards. Its energy helps surmount pesky irritations, the things that temporarily knock a person out of balance. It supplies the energy to meet challenges, especially deadlines or new situations. Lemon Grass energetically assists the development of patience and confidence.

The energy of Lemon Grass oil repairs holes in the auric field and protects the energy field from the bombardment of electromagnetic energy of radio, TV, computers, and other appliances. Lemon Grass oil also stimulates discernment to recognize the sources of discordant energy.

Using the oil for transformation

To feel discernment, use Lemon Grass to clear the solar plexus and sacral chakra. Add to massage oils for clearing the etheric body between the skin and the emotional body. Lemon Grass releases energy in the stomach meridian and digestive system. Take a bath in Lemon Grass oil to vitalize pranic energy to nourish the physical body.

Precautions

This oil is fairly non-irritating; to be certain check for a reaction.

LIME   *Citrus aurantifolia – Rutaceae*
Transformations

Key: Soothes Cellular Memories. Joy results from being totally cleansed and revitalized with Spiritual energy.

Growth and healing issues

Memories surface, indicating their need to become embraced into love, which heals and dissipates their density. Inappropriate energy attachments are disengaged.

Energetic influences on the bodies and chakras

Lime is a soothing salve to traumatic memories held in the etheric and physical bodies. Dense fearful emotions held in the cellular memory begin to release enabling conception of a new perception.

Energetics of the oil

Lime's refreshing sensation feels similar to the experience of rinsing the mouth out with fresh water after a salty ocean swim. The scent is a soothing salve to the etheric body. Energetically it cleanses traumatic emotions held in the cellular memory of the physical body. Using Lime creates a feeling of being totally cleansed and revitalized with Soul energy, a feeling of joy that expands into bliss and bubbles into the lightness of laughter.

Use Lime wherever body memory has begun to surface instead of trying to surface the actual memory. Sometimes the body is stuck in a time warp. When this happens scars and bruises from the past appear on the body. Lime oil helps to heal those scars and bring the body back into the present. Talk with your body, and tell it this experience is only a bleed-through from the past; this helps return the body to the present. Sometimes this memory is pain the inner child has experienced, and the child needs to become integrated with the present self to release the pain.

Use the oil with past-life therapy techniques. Lime is also a great oil to use for the Shamanic practice of cord-cutting. Cords are strings of energy attaching you to the physical and etheric bodies of other people, channeling energy and memories back and forth. Karmic cords can also be attached to people, places, and things. Cords drain off your energy. Massaging the oil into an attachment stimulates healing within the cellular memory.

Using the oil for transformation

Use the oil on any area that holds trauma to help soothe and release it out of the cellular memory.

Precautions

This oil is fairly non-irritating, to be certain check for a reaction. You can use more of this oil, 15-30 drops, in 2 ounces of a base oil. This oil can be photosensitizing; keep exposure to sunlight at a minimum. Citrus oils often have a high concentration of pesticides.

MARJORAM   *Origanum majorana – Labiatae*
Transformations

Key:Acknowledges Unconscious Fears. The ability to lovingly embrace the shadow self promotes an objective perspective, generating tremendous insight
to induce Spiritual growth. The heart's fear of vulnerability diminishes,
releasing the fear of being hurt, allowing greater joy into life and the learning of new responses.

Growth and healing issues

Feeling secure and connected to Spirit stimulates the desire to examine
fears. Spiritual growth progresses when the self examines and overcomes
unconscious reactions and behavior patterns. Greater responsibility and
control of your life empowers the personality and releases victim and dominator mentalities.

Energetic influences on the bodies and chakras

The root chakra expands and grounds energies, creating a greater foundation of security. The heart learns to stay open, which encourages feeling
comfortable and being present in the body. The third eye opens and aligns
with the Spiritual body, heightening intuition. The vibration increases, dis-
sipating density from the body and aura.

Energetics of the oil

Imagine yourself running through a field of blooming wildflowers.
Inhaling Marjoram oil recalls the joyful feelings and memories of being a
vivacious youth.

Marjoram's energy stimulates the recollection of many other types of
memories. Energetically, Marjoram supports feelings of security allowing
the recall of experiences attached to immense fear. It is an excellent energy to work with when recovering memories of abuse. Often the intensity
of abuse creates a need to be emotionally detached and in extreme cases,
the victim will develop a cold, aloof attitude. Marjoram creates a shift in
consciousness so that the experience aligns with the lesson's true purpose.
Learning the lesson allows a person to learn how to emotionally interact.

It then becomes possible to release the heart's energy from its state of separation and experience all the emotion that life has to offer.

On the physical level, Marjoram oil is a powerful anti-inflammatory. Experiencing joint pain and stiffness sometimes signals resistance or inflexibility of movement and thought. This rigidity is often a consequence of the fear of being a victim—to compensate the person needs to be in total control of everything. The "dominator" nature is marked by a headstrong conviction that their way is the only way. Often "their way" is the only way they know, but they assume it's their duty to straighten people out. Marjoram greatly helps symptoms arising from this type of energy.

Another factor behind a rigid personality is reliance upon external validation of self, as opposed to a more flexible person who has internal validation. Energetically Marjoram raises the vibration very quickly and brings density into alignment. Lightening density facilitates an alignment between spirit and matter so that change becomes easier. A stronger bond with the Higher Self generates greater self-esteem and self-reliance and relinquishes the need for validation from other people. Marjoram's rapid expansion of vibrational energy makes it easy to feel ungrounded, so combine Marjoram with a grounding oil.

Marjoram was a sacred plant to Shiva Vishnu in India, and it stimulates memories of past lives or the collective consciousness of India. Memories of Egypt are also stimulated, especially of the ancient times. During the Renaissance Marjoram had many therapeutic uses, and using the oil helps to unlock memories of life times spent in that period.

Using the oil for transformation

Massage the oil on the front and back of the throat and on the third eye. When the throat and third eye chakra are aligned, spiritual energy flows easily through the physical body. This energy allows you to move into higher frequencies of vibration. The front hollow of the ankle is the point that connects the dreaming or astral body to the physical body, Marjoram oil on that point grounds and balances energy coming into the body. Anointing the crown chakra and down to the base of the spine where the Kundalini energy coils stimulates the energy and enhances the spiritual alignment.

Marjoram is a good oil to rub on places where the body holds pain, especially arthritis. Use on joints for creating greater ease of movement. Inhaling the oil induces a wonderful dream state and provides relief to insomniacs.

Precautions

Avoid using during pregnancy. This oil is fairly non-irritating, to be certain check for a reaction. Use 15-30 drops in 2 ounces of a base oil. Be extra cautious when using this essential oil on children.

MYRRH GUM   *Commiphora myrrha – Burseraceae*
Transformations

Key: Releases Suffering and Sorrow. Realizing that love is the only protection needed allows walls and shields to dissipate. Learning to keep the heart open helps easily transmute difficult and painful experiences. Learning to be non-judgmental, accepting, and allowing energy to be what it is allows energy to flow unblocked and does not attract unneeded experiences.

Growth and healing issues

The martyr complex develops from a misguided need for the burdens of suffering and sorrow and maintains separation from Spirit. Not being true to Self drains spontaneity, creates anxiety, and obstructs joy. Blocked emotions create walls of density that separates one from emotional involvement and maintains separation from Spirit. Conforming to the confinement of the physical world discourages the perception of subtle energies. Developing norms dictated by Spirit produces energy to disengage from the mass consciousness reality, and releases notions restrictive of responsibility.

Energetic influences on the bodies and chakras

Being "out-of-body" means that the emotional, physical, mental, and etheric bodies are not integrated. One body can dominate over the others by determining what information is valid and ignoring input deemed invalid. Keeping the heart open helps one stay in the body. Self-trust produces an environment favorable to integration and allows more Spiritual energy to be manifested into the physical body.

Energetics of the oil

The unique scent of Myrrh feels haunting. Energetically it helps overcome the martyr's burden of suffering and sorrow.

The dysfunction of humanity and the chasm of separation from Source overwhelm people at times. Being caught up in the reality of mass consciousness disrupts a person's balance. Myrrh oil helps dispel the feelings of sorrow a person might feel about humanity's direction. Its energy helps an individual disengage from the mass consciousness conditioning. This is an important attribute of Myrrh because prescribed social reactions to emotional situations create a burdensome feeling of responsibility. Social norms also drain a person's spontaneous energy, obstructing the joy of being in the moment. Extended use of Myrrh Gum oil empowers a person to develop their norms guided by Source.

Using Myrrh Gum helps with issues of trust, especially the discovery of how much trust the self has in Self. To overcome blocks, a person must honestly look at what issues restrain their ability to trust. Intent coupled with the oil's gentle energy encourages looking at the fears that created the mistrust, and enable a person to admit to their loss of faith. Once resistance is acknowledged, trust in Self can begin rebuilding. Letting Spirit guide the way to the highest good promotes greater opportunity for Spiritual growth.

Constraining emotions causes a very dense and weary feeling. People believe that denying heart feelings protects them but it only achieves keeping them in a state of separation and furthers the spell of illusion. These denied emotions create walls of armor around the aura, which block the physical body's ability to receive replenishing Pranic energy. Dense walls around the aura make it feel uncomfortable to be in the body. Myrrh energy generates a feeling of being enveloped in a shield of love that reflects all harmful influences and lets the heart stay open. When a person is in an overwhelmed emotional state, Myrrh Gum oil gently eases anxious feelings by reopening the heart energy. Its soothing qualities bring the heart chakra into balance.

Using the oil for transformation

Myrrh Gum oil used on the heart area helps to keep it open in situations of stress. Stretch and massage the neck with Myrrh Gum oil to reduce mental tension and the need for control. This also releases issues of not trusting. To reduce anxiety, use the oil on the heart meridian. Using Myrrh Gum on the pericardium meridian helps to stimulate the feelings of protection and enhances intimacy.

Precautions

Avoid using during pregnancy. This oil is fairly non-irritating, to be certain check for a reaction. Use 15-30 drops in 2 ounces of a base oil.

MYRTLE   *Myrtus communis – Myrtaceae*
Transformations

Key: Comprehension of Energy Forms. Understanding the impermanent nature of matter resolves the conflict between the Soul's immortality and the personality's impatience. Past-life memories of practicing the ancient art of shape-shifting recall how to properly use and evoke power held in various forms.

Growth and healing issues

The male and female aspects come into balance, transforming their essences into a state of androgyny. Balancing the inner male and female traits facilitates the emergence into oneness, achieving harmony by resolving internal conflict and confusion. Recognizing the characteristics of various forms allows higher frequencies of light and love vibrations to assimilate.

Energetic influences on the bodies and chakras

Balancing male and female energies generates the ability to enact appropriate energy for any situation. The crown chakra aligns with all the chakras allowing dormant knowledge stored in each chakra to be used as a resource.

Energetics of the oil

Myrtle trees display the graceful beauty of both the male and female form contained within them. The energy of Myrtle brings the male and the female aspects into a state of balance, energetically melding the separate essences into a state of androgyny. Using Myrtle oil will help recall past lifetimes in the opposite gender.

Myrtle's essence helps us comprehend the consciousness of form and inspires appreciation of the grace and the beauty individual forms hold. This promotes remembrance of the ancient art of shapeshifting. Legends say shapeshifting was the magical skill of shifting consciousness or spirit into an animal, plant, or rock to unlock the secrets of that form's energy and knowledge. This comprehension of form Myrtle induces brings greater understanding about the changing nature of matter: that everything is cycling from one form into another. Myrtle initiates insights into immortality and the relationship between life and death. Myrtle's uses once included communicating with the dead. In the present, its energy would greatly aid in rebirthing therapies.

Myrtle oil helps assimilate higher vibrations of light. This assimilation facilitates awareness of a deep level of consciousness in all things—be they places, creatures, plants, animals, or inanimate objects. The vibrations promote a greater understanding of what it means to merge into oneness, as well as what it means to be truly individual.

Bible lore says God allowed Adam and Eve to take the Myrtle tree with them on their exodus from Eden. In Biblical times, Jewish women wore a wreath of Myrtle leaves to symbolize matrimony. Myrtle oil stimulates memories of Sumerian lifetimes for the Myrtle tree embodied the Sumerian Marienna, the Mother of Heaven. The Goddess Aphrodite also greatly loved the Myrtle tree and the energy of love is refined in the essence of the oil.

Using the oil for transformation

Massaging Myrtle oil into the pituitary reflex point of the foot helps move sluggish pituitary energy. Find the point in the center of the big toe and stimulate with firm pressure, while deep breathing. Rubbing the oil on the base of the skull also helps to stimulate memories.

To energize the spiritual body, massage the oil into the seventh cervical vertebra at the base of the neck and shoulders. This point aligns all the bodies' templates. Sometimes an individual experiences dimensional bleed-through, confusing their body about which reality it is presently in. To bring energy back into the present moment, massage the oil into the seventh vertebra while rocking the individual back and forth.

To begin learning shapeshifting, meditate with the oil and hold your intent on a specific issue or thing such as a crystal, geometric shape, or animal to draw in the power that they can unlock within.

Precautions

This oil is fairly non-irritating, to be certain check for a reaction. Use 15-30 drops in 2 ounces of a base oil.

NEROLI   *Citrus aurantium bigaradia — Rutaceae*
Transformations

Key: Encourages Self-Actualization. Developing inner trust increases self-acceptance and infuses the heart with self-actualization. A gentleness and vulnerability that encourages the heart to stay open through all experiences is instilled, producing feelings of security and protection.

Growth and healing issues

Invalidating feelings, self-pity, self-defeating attitudes, and low self-esteem all contribute to fragmentation of the self. Embracing self in love reunites the fragmented parts into a state of wholeness. This increases inner trust, inner faith, and generates the inner strength necessary to become self-actualized. Issues surrounding women's menses often caused by frustration, criticism, and anger directed inward can be resolved with a new attitude.

Energetic influences on the bodies and chakras

Male and female aspects of the heart are opened and balanced. The reproductive organs and chakras feel nurtured by the energy. The emotional, mental, and physical bodies overcome inner turmoil and confusion when the energy of self-love is directed inwards.

Energetics of the oil

The energy of Neroli is like a loving parental hug given to a child after a painful fall. Neroli opens and balances the female and male aspects of the heart bringing feelings of security, protection, and an intense feeling of being loved to all aspects of self. Neroli brings the heart into the vulnerable state, a very feminine feeling of opening up to the world, and balances it with the masculine aspects of taking control of life.

Invalidating self causes great harm to the emotional, mental, and physical bodies and results in fragmenting self. Neroli helps validate feelings. Its uplifting scent dispels self-pity and self-defeating attitudes, and empowers the self with inner strength and faith. Valuing feelings develops a deeper inner trust, allowing greater self-acceptance. Energetically, Neroli oil reunites and integrates all aspects of self for actualizing on the physical plane.

Neroli also helps relieve menstrual cramps. Often women have a difficult time dealing with their menses because they are not taught to celebrate their female body, but to be critical of it. Women direct their frustration and criticism inwards, which creates confusion within the female organs. This could lead serious problems in the future, such as endometriosis, ovarian cysts, or other female organ dysfunction. The menses are a cycle of purification and should be a celebration of Nature's rhythms, but are usually only celebrated as a sign of not being pregnant.

Neroli oil stimulates memories of lifetimes in Spain and Morocco. Many brides wore the Neroli blossoms in their hair as symbols of purity and fertility. The flower represented the energy of the Virgin Mary. The white flower is symbolic of her virginity and the fruit symbolic of the chastity of her labor.

Using the oil for transformation

Using Neroli on the root chakra and pubic bone grounds the feminine form into the physical. Release depression by using the oil on the solar plexus.

Neroli on the heart area helps to balance heart energy. Rub inside the wrist to calm tension and anxiety held in the emotional body.

Massaging Neroli oil on the conception and governing meridians helps to ground and energize the life force. Using the oil on the pericardium, conception, and spleen meridians help with menstrual discomfort. Ground the male energy of taking control of life by massaging the oil into the liver meridian. Open feminine energy for expressing love energy by using the oil on the heart meridian. Massaging the small intestine meridian with the oil helps to differentiate feelings of impurity and purity, release self-judgment, and promote greater feelings of self worth. When you are socializing, dab the oil on the wrists and behind the ears to attract people to you and to give you courage in crowds.

Precautions

Be suspicious of this oil's purity because it is often diluted with synthetics or less expensive constituents. Citrus oils often have a high concentration of pesticides. This oil is fairly non-irritating, to be certain check for a reaction. Dilute 15-30 drops in 2 ounces of a base oil.

NUTMEG   Myristica fragrans – Myristicaceae
Transformations

Key: Eases Betrayal and Loss, Increases Flexibility and Spontaneity. Understanding the impermanence of life allows flexibility and the ability to be happy wherever you are. Cultivating the attitude that life is an adventure full of wonderful surprises lets traveling or moving (emotionally, mentally, or physically) to become second nature. This attitude facilitates abundance by encouraging a sense of liberation that diminishes limitation. Inner-strength develops from flexibility and detachment.

Growth and healing issues

When the heart is allowed to dance with Spirit, the constraints of rigidity and permanence that suppress joyful spontaneity are released. Shifting the attitude from loss to an opportunity builds new foundations and the ability to more easily soothe the feelings stimulated by severing an attachment that contributes to feelings of self-doubt and pessimism. An appropriate grieving period provides the space to release the old and prepare to begin anew.

Energetic influences on the bodies and chakras

The heart learns to stay open through times of emotional anguish produced by the shattering of an illusion. The solar plexus receives comforting energy when experiencing tremendous emotional and mental turmoil caused by the perception of betrayal and deception. The root chakra learns to maintain a grounded state, enabling greater flexibility in change.

Energetics of the oil

The energy of Nutmeg oil unleashes the wild free spirit within and encourages the heart to dance with joy. Nutmeg's energy recalls the feelings of a warm, loving, and jovial family gathering. Use Nutmeg in the gloomy wintertime to lighten the spirit. Nutmeg supports you when you must rebuild your life or rebirth your self.

Energetically, Nutmeg oil inspires the desire to overcome the burden of rigidity and liberate the Spirit. Nutmeg connects you with the wild and free nature within you, the place from which abundance emanates. It is useful for people who are moving or traveling because it inspires inner happiness and comfort where ever they are. Nutmeg energetically cultivates carefree and transient energy, overcoming sedentary feelings and limitations by expanding feeling to the immensity of potential. This expanded energy repels permanence and inflexibility to change. Meditating with the oil illuminates the meaning of immortality.

Nutmeg oil is also excellent for people who have moved a lot and feel as if they have missed something by not having roots. Working with Nutmeg subdues feelings of loss, especially those created by a missed opportunity or fearing a wrong decision was made. Nutmeg reminds us there is no right or wrong, only the need to experience. The sense of loss is an internally creat-ed frustration. Nothing can be truly lost, only hidden from self.

Nutmeg oil's energy comforts the anguish of losing sentimental pos-sessions. Energetically it helps with the grief stemming from the cata-strophic loss incurred in a fire, flood, or other disaster. It helps shift the density of loss into the motivated energy needed to rebuild. Nutmeg helps lift the emotional body to a state of detachment, an understanding that material possessions don't matter on the journey of life and memories are all you need to carry.

Nutmeg comforts people feeling rejected and betrayed in affairs of the heart by easing the sharp, constricting pain felt in the gut and heart. The feeling of dying inside is actually constricting bands of energy around the heart. Nutmeg shatters illusions of relationships and lets truth be seen, allowing closure to a relationship.

Nutmeg brings comfort and support to people who feel the dark around them or who have fallen into an intense black hole of emotion. Using the oil helps transform the feelings of pessimism and hopelessness that oppress the Spirit, letting them perceive a brighter future. Nutmeg also helps lighten up the energy of a person who is taking himself too seriously.

The Nutmeg tree is native to the West Indies and can recall memories of the early colonization of the New World. Nutmeg embodies the arche-typal energy of trading and pirates.

Using the oil for transformation

Not feeling supported in life creates lower back pain; a massage with Nutmeg oil will help alleviate the pain. Nutmeg energy works to cleanse the pancreas, which constricts from lack of joy in life. It also stimulates the appetite and is especially helpful for those people who have a hard time assimilating food, a sign they are not receiving nourishment from life. Nutmeg is a good morn-ing oil because of its invigorating energy but it may cause insomnia if used at night. Nutmeg can be hallucinogenic so be careful and limit the use.

Precautions

Do not use this oil on children or infants. Avoid using during pregnancy. Overuse of Nutmeg oil can cause headaches. Nutmeg oil can irritate the skin and mucous membranes. Dilute 1-10 drops in 2 ounces of a base oil before applying to the skin. Use only 1-5 drops in a bath.

ORANGE (SWEET)   *Citrus aurantium sinensis – Rutaceae*

Transformations

Key: Releases Density from the Aura. Developing an attitude of non-judgmental allowance maintains balance during life's challenges and encourages staying centered and true to your Spirit.

Growth and healing issues

Detaching from the intensity of drama dissolves unknown fears and obsessions and promotes a more objective perspective; highly charged emotions are calmed. Clearing the aura and environment of disharmonious energies prevents attracting similar dense and uncomfortable vibrations or entities.

Energetic influences on the bodies and chakras

Expelling negativity, entities, and dense thought forms repairs the aura. The astral body also benefits by clearing the residue of a night of traveling through the astral planes.

Energetics of the oil

Sweet Orange has an uplifting and calming feeling, like being thrown a lifesaver after falling into a sea of emotion. This oil releases negativism (density) from the auric field. It also dispels negative thought patterns, especially those from entities—which can be collective thoughts—resonating in a person's living and work space.

Orange oil repairs rips in the auric field that create energy leaks. The oil also helps relieve obsessions by transforming them into states of allowance. Orange oil aides dream therapy by stimulating the astral body, which can provide answers to many unknown fears and tensions. Keeping a dream journal while using Orange energy creates an insightful tool for discovering the unconscious issues affecting your life.

Using the oil for transformation

Sweet orange placed on the solar plexus and second chakra helps repair the energy field. Massage the oil on the physical body, especially the spleen area, whenever an energy drain is felt or unconsciously acknowledged. When massaging on the spleen rub vigorously in an up and down motion, this seals the energy from possible disruptions from outside influences.

Energetically, Orange purifies the highly charged emotional vibrations that remain in physical spaces after an event has passed. Spray or burn this oil in the air to clear those areas, for instance, spray in an area after an argument to release the hot emotion. Clearing the area frees up the energy field of your work or living space.

Anointing the wrist brings a calming feeling; holding the points on the outsides of the wrist relieves hysteria. A bath with Orange oil after an argument also produces a calming effect.

Precautions

This oil can be slightly irritating to the skin and potentially sensitizing; check for a reaction. Dilute 15-20 drops of oil in 2 ounces of base oil. Keep exposure to sunlight at a minimum when using this oil because it can be photosensitizing. Be extra cautious when using this essential oil on children. Citrus oils often have a high concentration of pesticides.

PALMAROSA   *Cymbopogon martinii—Graminaceae*

Transformations

Key: Comprehends Divine Mother Energy. Establishes compassionate acceptance and unconditional love by generating a higher frequency of Spiritual Love. Greater understanding of being a mother or of relationship dynamics with a mother is gained. Healing our Mother issues allows us to become more self-sufficient and be better mothers to ourselves.

Growth and healing issues

Energy distortions or issues arising from your relationship with your mother are realized and the healing process begins. Palmarosa energetically helps us recognize the role models we use for creating relationships and promotes discovery of the motives and roles we act out within the family dynamics. The core issue in all relationships is often based upon lack of self-love and the tendency to fill that lack with a substitution.

Energetic influences on the bodies and chakras

Calms the nervous system and helps overcome the need to be perfect. Generates more acceptance and appreciation for your current physical form. Opens a greater receptivity to nurturing by Mother Earth.

Energetics of the oil

Palmarosa establishes compassionate acceptance and unconditional love. Energetically the oil invokes Mother energy—the ability to birth life into existence, be it a baby, relationship, or a creative endeavor. It generates the higher frequency of Spiritual Love and reveals inherent knowledge of the principles of manifestation. The oil opens us to the nurturing of Mother Earth. Understanding the true role of motherhood encourages us to value the life spark in all existence and to recognize our oneness.

A mother is the vehicle through which we manifest into the physical. It is our deepest bond with another human. Our interaction with our mothers is the model we use when creating other relationships. Palmarosa oil is excellent to use when the bond with your mother has developed a distorted pattern. Energetically, Palmarosa heals feelings of abandonment and of not being loved by our birth mother. Palmarosa stimulates Spiritual mother energy that nourishes our inner child. Using the oil during regression therapy stimulates greater healing of issues arising from a dysfunctional relationship with our mothers. Healing mother issues allows you to learn to become a mother to yourself, which generates all-encompassing love towards self and allows you to receive spiritual nurturing from the

Soul. This oil could also be beneficial to adopted individuals with issues of not knowing their birth mother.

Energetically Palmarosa oil helps to change the dynamics between mother and child, enabling more appropriate bonds to be created or renewed. We often believe our mother is the cause of our problems in life. Palmarosa energy reminds us that we are responsible for our lack of self-esteem, that we chose our parents and the lessons we wanted to learn through the family relationship. Mothers are called upon to act out certain roles we agreed upon before embodying into the physical to help us learn a lesson or experience a specific energy. Mothers also ask that their children teach them specific lessons. Perceiving it in this way begins to heal the dysfunctional relationship and supports embracing the relationship in love.

Palmarosa anchors appreciation for the wonder of creation and enhances reverence for the physical form. Using the oil while meditating on our love/hate relationship with our physical form allows us to love our bodies more fully. We understand the reason for being in the physical, and feel appreciation and acceptance of it and learn to live more fully and harmoniously in our physical bodies. When we live more fully in our bodies we can manifest more Spiritual energy onto the planet. The true essence of motherhood—for women and for men—is to manifest energy into physical form.

Using the oil for transformation

Palmarosa has an affinity with the air, stimulating the Higher Mind to perceive visions of the future. Using the oil on the triple warmer and conception meridians can enhance loving the physical form. Use the oil on the stomach meridian and colon region to learn to let go. Anointing the heart and pericardium meridians will allow greater intimacy to be felt.

Precautions

Be suspicious of this oil's purity because it is often diluted with synthetics or less expensive constituents. This oil is fairly non-irritating, to be certain check for a reaction. Dilute 15-30 drops in 2 ounces of a base oil.

PATCHOULI   *Pogostemon cablin – Labiatae*
Transformations

Key: Grounds and Fortifies the Will to Live. Developing a reverent attitude towards the sacredness of life generates an appreciation of learning through life's challenges and strengthens the connection with Spirit. Questioning established beliefs expands consciousness and affirms the desire to change and grow.

Growth and healing issues

Not having a strong connection to the Earth creates distortions in the root chakra's energy, which hinders nurturing from the healing forces of nature. Grounding into the physical and living in the present releases depression and suicidal thoughts.

Energetic influences on the bodies and chakras

Unlocking the root and sacral chakras' sexual issues helps align their energy to the heart chakra. The fears of survival in those chakras are resolved by increasing faith in Spirit. Being grounded into the physical produces the energy necessary to take action.

Energetics of the oil

Patchouli energy creates an affinity with the heartbeat of Mother Nature. It embodies the feeling of being cradled in her arms and immersed in the Earth's essence. Patchouli has a very grounding capacity.

Energetically Patchouli oil heightens reverence for life, an attitude that honors the value of all life experiences and all life forms and accepts that a spark of sacredness exists in all matter. Reverence is not the same as respect, which is a judgment about qualities we admire, but a perception of life as the school for spiritual development. When we lack reverence we perceive experiences with judgment. Striving for reverence makes us protective of all life and aligns us with Soul energy.

Patchouli oil dispels the blues. Patchouli oil opens the root chakra, helping us ground in the present moment and surrender to just being. It helps us feel more joy in our physical form and face responsibilities.

Patchouli oil expands the life force outward, further anchoring the Spirit into the physical. Energetically, it is a powerful oil for overcoming suicidal tendencies. Its energy enhances the will to live.

Patchouli oil's essence unlocks the sacral chakra's sensual energy and transforms states of frigidity into sensuality. It allows greater understanding of intimate relations with other people. This is spiritual energy as well as sexual—Patchouli aligns the root and sacral chakras with the energy of the heart chakra.

Patchouli was popular in the Sixties, a time of great experimental consciousness and questioning established beliefs. Many doorways to reality were explored by those pioneering New Age thought. Marijuana was used as a means of stimulating awareness. Patchouli oil's rise in popularity was due to an unconscious desire to ground the effects of the pot. In many cultures throughout history and still today drugs are sacred tools for opening the doorways of perception.

Using the oil for transformation

Patchouli oil feels wonderful when massaged into the stomach meridian, balancing the Earth element within and sending forth greater nourishment of self love. Massage the intestine reflex points of the hands and feet to further stimulate the Earth energy. Massaging Patchouli on the bridge of the nose and brow helps to alleviate depression. Use the oil on the spleen and gall bladder meridians to bring a person into balance with joy. Use the oil on the kidney meridian for help with being in the moment. Do deep breathing while inhaling the Patchouli oil and focus your intent to be completely in your physical body with your heart open. Extend the energy of the light body out and notice how different it feels. Also use on the heart, root and sacral chakras to align sensuality. Massage into the root and sacral chakras to heal suicidal thoughts.

Precautions

This oil is fairly non-irritating, to be certain check for a reaction. Dilute 15-30 drops in 2 ounces of a base oil.

PENNYROYAL   *Mentha pulegium — Lamiaceae (Labiatae)*
Transformations

Key: Heals Solar Plexus Distortions. Recognizing mass consciousness beliefs supports disconnecting from it and training your intent to establish and support new truths as your reality. The energy heightens intuition and creativity.

Growth and healing issues

Pennyroyal oil extends a protective influence over those prone to negativity or easily overwhelmed by increased amounts of sensory information. Its energy forms a protective shield against psychic projections. The passions of possessiveness and jealousy resolve when trust in Self increases.

Energetic influences on the bodies and chakras

Distortions in solar plexus energy begin to heal, clarifying and resolving emotional and mental body confusion. Decision-making is made easier by calming mind chatter. Soul energy is more firmly anchored into the physical body.

Energetics of the oil

The scent of Pennyroyal penetrates deep into the solar plexus, summoning vitality to the emotional and mental bodies. Energetically, Pennyroyal oil clears the mind, easing confusion created by constant mental chatter. Chatter leads to self-doubt and clouds decision-making. Judgment and resistance allows negativity to saturate the emotional and mental bodies. Pennyroyal assists in repelling negative thought forms by disconnecting you from overwhelming mass consciousness. Clearing the solar plexus chakra engages the ability to discriminate the origins of energy and establishes a strong and healthy sense of individuality.

Pennyroyal expands the aura by anchoring the Soul into the physical body. Be careful with Pennyroyal—too much will so highly accelerate energy transference that it can make you dizzy or nauseous. The physical body does not adjust quickly enough to assimilate and ground the energy and the Soul must reduce itself to partake in the human experience, much like electricity goes through transformers to be compatible with the current an appliance needs.

The oil's energy overcomes the passions of possessiveness and jealousy by forging a stronger bond with the Higher Self. Obsessive attachments to people, places, and material things are attributes of the personality's feeling a lack of power. When personality is infused with Source, the need to have power over others becomes unnecessary and is released by self-fulfillment and a greater trust of intuition.

Using the oil for transformation

Pennyroyal inspires artistic creativity in the psyche by strengthening the bond with the Soul. Its energy protects the aura, especially when a person is in an ungrounded expanded state of creativity. Its energy protects novice travelers of the astral world, where it is possible to fall into negative states of mind. It permits negative energy to flow uninhibited through the aura without attaching or dragging down a person's energy. Pennyroyal protects a person's energy field from psychic projections by embracing those projections and closing any opportunity to hook into the aura. Pennyroyal supports ritual Shamanic cord cutting, a technique to release energy attachments. This same energy, however, is detrimental to woman who are pregnant or trying to conceive. It hinders a baby's soul from attaching and bonding with the mother and may cause miscarriage.

Precautions

Avoid using during pregnancy and never use the oil internally as an abortive—it is highly toxic and could be fatal taken internally. Do not use this oil on children or infants. This oil is fairly non-irritating, to be certain check for a reaction. Dilute 15-30 drops in 2 ounces of a base oil.

PEPPERMINT   *Mentha piperita – Labiatae*
Transformations

Key: Activates the Higher-Mind. The inner sight understands and interprets the consciousness represented in geometric and symbolic forms. Accessing the Higher Mind heightens intuition and permits communication with the consciousness of other life forms. Being receptive to messages originating in the universal mind builds new foundations of reality from Soul-infused truths.

Growth and healing issues

Peppermint energy cools the friction of resistance to new information. The Higher Mind calms memories of terror, hysteria, and fear of the unknown, which hinder growth by surfacing their cause and diminishing their emotional charge.

Energetic influences on the bodies and chakras

Unblocking stagnant energy in the etheric body allows assimilation and balance of physical energy and calms the terror sometimes experienced when the light body shifts. Grounding this increased Spiritual energy into physical action is facilitated by dialogue with the personality, emotional, and mental bodies.

Energetics of the oil

The scent of Peppermint evokes remembrance of a day filled with kaleidoscope color and crispness in the air. It has an autumn quality to its energy recalling the harvest period. Energetically the oil is a key that can unlock the gift for understanding symbols originating in the Higher Mind. It has a mythological association with Griffins, the guardians of treasure.

Peppermint energy opens that part of mind that conveys thought by generating symbols or geometric forms. Peppermint's energy reveals the universal consciousness held in these forms, which supports learning the language of Nature and other life forms. Peppermint expands the third eye chakra and aligns its energy with the first chakra, actualizing a grounded spiritual energy into physical action. The mental body is balanced and infused with Soul knowledge. The oil works on a variety of issues that energetically dissolve the mental body's fears, calms mind chatter and clears confusion.

Peppermint oil is a great aide to the stomach and symbolically helps digestion of new thoughts and beliefs. Energetically, Peppermint oil helps create a new foundation of reality based on our inner light or Soul energy.

Dealing with the rapid change of reality can cause symptoms experienced as cramps and pains in the legs. When moving through changes in energies, the legs have a tendency to become blocked and Peppermint can alleviate this type of pain. It works on the etheric body, allowing the energy to flow down into the physical.

Peppermint oil will help to cool heat in the body caused by friction of resisting energy. Use the oil at night when the strong energies that produce night sweats can come into the dreaming body. Peppermint cools menopausal hot flash symptoms and alleviates the intense pain of a migraine headache, especially those headaches caused by a clashing of spiritual and physical energy.

Its use has roots in Britain where it was used to create a wall between the dimensions separating us from the Brownies, Gnomes, and other fairy folk. Back then the little people inspired fear and people did not want them around. If you are experiencing chaotic energy in your environment that you think might be caused by mischievous "little people," peppermint can dissuade their impish presence. Peppermint does not grow proficiently in gardens with a high population of Nature Spirits. Ask the Nature Spirits not to interpret the Peppermint as a sign to stay away. In ancient Egypt, the herb was associated with the god Horus, and was said to embody the energy of protection and wisdom.

Using the oil for transformation

Use on the temples for soothing comfort to headaches. A compress of vinegar helps release the toxins creating the symptom. Inhaling peppermint is uplifting and energizing and clears stress lodged in the mental body. It opens the sinuses expanding the crown chakra and deepens the ability to breathe, bringing in a greater desire to live. Peppermint on the spleen and liver meridians relieves menstrual cramps. Do not inhale at night for it might cause insomnia, but use as a lotion rubbed on the body on a hot night for its cooling actions. Use peppermint tea to settle the stomach and rub oil on the stomach and intestine meridians to open any energy blocks and aid in the ability to let go. Placing the oil on the soles of the feet and the crown chakra and visualizing the energy running up and down the bodies several times breaks up any stagnation held in the etheric bodies and reduces any terror felt within the physical body as light body expands.

Precautions

This oil is fairly non-irritating, to be certain check for a reaction. Use 15-30 drops in 2 ounces of a base oil. Never use undiluted peppermint oil to massage the total body, it has a chilling effect that feels unpleasantly like being encased in a block of ice. Peppermint oil reduces the effectiveness of homeopathic remedies.

PETITGRAIN   *Citrus aurantium var. amara —Rutaceae*
Transformations

Key: Overcomes Obsessions and Addictions. Understanding issues that arise from power struggles and the need to control and taking responsibility for self and your reality weakens an addiction's control over the personality. Generating more self-love and self-acceptance nurtures and fills the lack behind addiction.

Growth and healing issues

The energy helps acknowledge and overcome obsessive and addictive behavioral patterns. Numbing self from the anguish of life, and feeling the shame of not taking responsibility for one's power and actions, often contributes to addictive behaviors. Liberation from addictions requires reintegration of the self, which resolves internal conflicts and the need for rationalizing behavior.

Energetic influences on the bodies and chakras

Petitgrain oil helps physical grounding and strengthens the desire to live, which helps overcome addictions. Shame held in the mental body eases when it is embraced into love. All addictions distort heart energy and often rip holes in the aura, which are repaired by loving the self.

Energetics of the oil

Petitgrain recalls the ominous feeling of walking through a forest, aware of a presence lurking around the fringes. Energetically, Petitgrain oil address-es addictions and obsessive behaviors. The oil imparts awareness of the patterns of numbing the self from anguish. Petitgrain energy dissolves the tension of issues that feel very painful to accept even to admit to self.

Addictions are characterized by overwhelming desire or fear and behavior that can not be satiated. There are many types of addiction: in addition to the obvious ones there are gossip, negative thought, drama, risk taking, dishonesty, always being busy, overworking, and constant talking. All are forms of avoidance and denial. All of these behaviors are created by either control or power issues.

The only way to effectively overcome an addiction is to acknowledge the true cause, which takes honest introspection. The personality often rationalizes the presence of an addiction, which is its resistance to Soul. We know the personality resists change, and knows that recovery from addic-tion means changing basic life premises. Diligent probing into how an addiction serves the personality leads to understanding the motivation. When the true cause comes into awareness it can be embraced into the heart and loved. Fearing and judging the addiction reinforces the behavior; it is only possible to change the habit by loving that part of self generating the behavior. Once the parts of self in conflict are identified, you can dialogue with them and ask them to integrate into wholeness.

Many opportunities will tempt you back into the habit, but if you back-slide be gentle and tell yourself you choose not to again. Do not give up or judge your self as a failure but keep your intent focused and move in that direction. Each time you overcome temptation you are stronger, and it is important to acknowledge your growth. One day it will not be a struggle or even perceived as a temptation; it will be your choice.

Petitgrain grounds the physical body, which aids in overcoming addic-tive behavior. Its energy opens the solar plexus chakra establishing the strength to take responsibility and to set boundaries. This also imparts a sense of being in control, which helps to subdue obsessive behaviors and instills assertiveness and the ability to make choices.

Different substances affect different chakras in diverse ways, blocking, disrupting, or distorting energy flow in the body and between chakras. All addictions ultimately arise when the heart closes and distorts heart chakra energy. After addiction cravings subside the chakras and aura must be repaired or the individual will find another substitution. An addict needs self-love to totally heal.

Using the oil for transformation

Applying on crown and brow chakras stimulates clarity of mental energy. Massaging the liver and gallbladder meridian points on the head and temples relieves mental tension. Rubbing into colon, liver, and gallbladder area releases the emotional energy of self-pity. Massaging the liver meridian helps to release states of denial. Stroking the oil into the stomach meridian encourages self-acceptance. Use on the kidney meridian helps to overcome fear of the future, enabling a person to live in the moment.

Massaging oil into the base of the skull and holding the prominent bony points of the occiput (found at the base of the head where the neck connects) stimulates repressed memory. Use on the medial aspect of the inside calf muscle about a fourth of the way down from the knee. This point feels very tender, especially in people who overextend themselves.

Precautions

This oil is fairly non-irritating, to be certain check for a reaction. Use 15-30 drops in 2 ounces of a base oil. Citrus oils often have a high concentration of pesticides.

PINE   *Pinus sylvestris – Coniferae*
Transformations

Key: *Awareness of Group Consciousness.* Group consciousness aspires towards enlightenment. It anchors the desire for living in community, an environment that provides for growth and nurturing. Groups will be structured to allow members to perform tasks using their talents in harmony with their Spiritual purpose.

Growth and healing issues

Helps to realize the traits or behaviors that hinder group consciousness from being actualized. Issues of separation, pride, humility, and ego control are replaced with knowing that we belong to and are part of a greater whole. Isolation and loneliness are warmed by the fellowship of others on the Spiritual path. Competition, alienation, and suspicion will dissipate as group members support each other and share vision. The challenge for loners is to learn how to receive nurturing from the group and release patterns of being nurtured by seclusion.

Energetic influences on the bodies and chakras

Pine energy allows greater self-expression by aligning the throat, third eye, sacral, and root chakras. The root chakra will expand in the supportive environment, intensifying the will to live. Living in a supportive environment opens the heart.

Energetics of the oil

The scent of Pine brings associations of wintertime festivals and awakens memories of warm social interaction. Energetically Pine oil stimulates introspection. The pinecone lies dormant; awaiting the season of germination, like seeds placed in the collective consciousness anticipating the emergence of new paradigms.

Pine energy spurs a cohesive group consciousness aspiring to enlightenment. The pinecone is a metaphor of group consciousness—just as all the seeds live in individuality within the structure of the cone, so each member holds in mind the intent of the group. Each individual member performs a function within the group that fulfills their unique Spiritual purpose while creating a healthy interdependence with others. Each contributes their excellence and resistance dissolves in fulfillment and joy. Through this cohesion, a greater concentration of energy is focused, manifesting a reality harmonious to all involved. Meditating in the Pine trees with the oil helps begin the process of visualizing the new form of life that the group can sustain.

Pine oil also transforms ego pride, which hinders working within a group. Pride maintains separation and impedes group consciousness. Pine oil has a two-fold effect on pride: it softens pompous pride in those needing constant external validation by infusing Spiritual purpose, and it increases pride in those suffering from a low self-esteem or small self-image.

Using the oil for transformation

Use Pine on tight neck muscles to loosen the mental body's need for control over the physical body. Massage the oil on the heart and pectoral muscles to release the tension held in that area. Massaging Pine oil into the abdomen releases the stress of ego control from the etheric solar plexus. Rub the oil on the front hollows of the collarbone to release detrimental thoughts and criticisms taken to heart. The gallbladder and liver channels benefit from Pine's cleansing and purifying effect. Rubbing Pine onto the stomach channel and abdomen releases anti-social behaviors and allows group consciousness to be grasped. Dissipate stagnant energy by using Pine on the soles of the feet, especially on the colon points around the heels. This also increases physical stamina. Using Pine oil on the bladder meridian generates supportive and encouraging feelings that help manifesting the group consciousness. To promote a greater cohesion of group consciousness, stimulate the heart and pericardium meridians with Pine oil's energy, releasing old fears of intimate relationships with others allowing deeper emotions and experiences of love.

Precautions

Pine oil is often diluted with turpentine. This oil can be slightly irritating to the skin and potentially sensitizing; check for a reaction. Dilute 15-20 drops of oil in 2 ounces of base oil.

ROSE   *Rosa spp. – Rosaceae*
Transformations

Key: Comprehending the Individuality of Oneness Allows the Experience of True Unconditional Love. The many different forms of the Rose acknowledge humanity's co-creative involvement in the Plant Kingdom's evolution, and humanity's divine role of stewardship. Infusing the personality with tenderness instills inner peace and lets the creativity of the Soul shine through the personality.

Growth and healing issues

Deeper intimacy in a relationship is achieved by examining fears underlying possessiveness, jealousy, or neediness. Not trusting a partner is incompatible with establishing an environment of true unconditional love. Acceptance and understanding are qualities of Divine Love that promote self-love.

Energetic influences on the bodies and chakras

Male and female energies are balanced. Rose energy has a tremendous ability to open the heart. Acknowledging that everything is a form of Spirit stimulates love for everything. The crown chakra expands, accessing new paradigms that will allow new realities to flourish.

Energetics of the oil

The energy of Rose is like seeing a rainbow after a deluge. The Rose is unique among flowers in its sheer variety. Each rainbow of color emanates a different frequency. Each rose has its own name, exemplifying the individual in its evolution. The development of hybrid roses is an excellent example of Humanity's co-creative involvement furthering the evolution of the Plant Kingdom. Roses grow in a lush variety of shapes, hues, and fragrances, all exquisitely beautiful. The spiraling petal around the center of the Rose bud resembles a chakra, and the bud opening into blossom is analogous to the opening of a chakra's energy.

Rose petals represent qualities of gentleness and softness, whereas the thorn represents the walls built around the emotions for protection. The energy of Rose engages softness within an individual who has a thorny personality by conveying the protection that Spirit provides. This protective energy dissolves the defense mechanisms that guard against emotional hurt. Male and female qualities are both inherent to the Rose form and energy. The feminine attributes are reflected in the Rose's gentleness, grace, and beauty, while the male traits are reflected in the thorns' protection and strength. This dual nature of the Rose balances male and female energy. The Rose is loved and worn by both sexes, projecting an elegance of dignity to both.

Rose cries the tears of humanity, and lends its assistance to transmuting the burden humanity carries. Sometimes Rose energy feels suffocating because it exposes the collective consciousness of the Piscean Age. Rose energy creates awareness of the crystallization and limitation of the beliefs of mass consciousness. It prompts Self to realize its extensive attachment to that reality, allowing Self to disengage from those unconscious thought patterns. The Piscean belief of suffering and salvation absolves by calling upon Divine Grace. Rose energy brings Divine Love and Grace into your life.

Divine Love is an attribute of Rose energy. If you have resisted love, meditate with Rose oil for insights into the issues that inhibit receiving affection and intimacy. Rose oil can open and expand the heart energy. Energetically it is one of the most powerful heart openers on the planet. It is appropriate to use Rose oil to focus on relationship issues. Rose energy surfaces awareness of clinging neediness and jealousy patterns, and diminishes these oppressive feelings that result from low self-esteem and distrusting self. Divine Grace transforms those patterns by energetically strengthening your relationship with Self, producing feelings of inner peace and self-reliance.

One way the unconscious mind communicates with the conscious mind is through dream symbols. The Rose, with its long association with human creation, is a prevalent dream symbol. Seeing a red rose represents a message from a Master, and if the dreamer received the rose, it means an etheric healing is possible. A white rose can signify a blessing from Jesus or indicate the presence of Archangel Raphael, whereas the red rose heralds Archangel Gabriel's presence. A pink rose proclaims assistance coming from the Saints, and the yellow rose symbolizes a covenant made between disciples on the journey of Spirit. Wild roses suggest that the dreamer renew self with Nature. A crown of thorns informs the presence of Jesus and that a spiritual alignment is to occur.

Rose energy promotes both outer and inner health and beauty. Cosmetically Rose softens the skin, renewing and regenerating the cells. Rose water refreshes tired eyes. Rose hips, the fruit of the rose, are high in vitamin C. On the etheric level, Rose fortifies inner strength by exposing the inner beauty, and budding it out into the physical plane.

Using the oil for transformation

Massage Rose oil along the liver meridian to encourage the development of responsibility. Rose clears obstructions in the liver meridian that hinder self-assertiveness. Rose releases energy blocks in the liver and lung meridians, helping you overcome feelings of guilt, sorrow, and self-righteousness. Using Rose on the kidney and spleen meridians awakens the determination to accomplish goals. Massaging Rose oil on the bladder meridian helps you relinquish the need to carry the burden of the mass consciousness. Rose oil massaged on the triple warmer meridian releases old patterns of behavior to allow new relationships to develop. Use Rose oil at night to call forth dreams.

You will experience the gentleness of the rose when inhaling its fragrance. Energetically, Rose releases old realities and thought forms and the process can feel like waves of energy moving out of the aura.

It takes tons of petals to produce one ounce of Rose oil. Most of the Rose oil on the market is very expensive unless it is synthetic. The synthetic oil has a different frequency as that of Rose absolute. If the absolute is too expensive, use fresh-cut roses. Meditating with cut roses is good though the energy fades fast. You could grow roses in your garden, but you might find it very hard to stop at just one variety.

Precautions

Be suspicious of this oil's purity because it is often diluted with synthetics or less expensive constituents. This oil is fairly non-irritating, to be certain check for a reaction. Use 15-30 drops in 2 ounces of a base oil.

ROSEMARY   *Rosmarinus officinalis – Labiatae*

Transformations

Key: Realizing True Loyalty. Being faithful to one's truth fortifies self-esteem and purpose. True loyalty connects the heart with the Soul. Spiritual love frees you from maintaining the state of lack and increases the ability to nourish Self. Generating more self-love heals and restores fragmented parts of Self to wholeness and innocence. To love another you need to love self first.

Growth and healing issues

The energy of loyalty to others may promote or constrict Spiritual growth and create karma; identifying motive indicates whether loyalties are appropriate or not. Bringing closure to a relationship eases feelings of grief, loneliness, and abandonment caused by heartbreak. Realizing and embracing the root-cause helps to overcome obsessions that contribute to insecurity and codependent behaviors. Embracing shortcomings allows the choice to react consciously. Transforming feelings of betrayal and shame allows incest survivors to create new attitudes and increase self-esteem.

Energetic influences on the bodies and chakras

The heart expands and feels soothed; the mental body relaxes. Cellular memories of abuse and incest can safely release when the memories are detached from charged emotions. Releasing grief and heartbreak allows lung energy to expand and nourish the body.

Energetics of the oil

Rosemary means "dew of the sea." Rosemary was traditionally used at both weddings and funerals. Its energy represents the dichotomy of love and death.

Energetically, Rosemary oil helps us recognize issues surrounding loyalty and love. Blind loyalty has a tendency to restrict energy, making you miss opportunities to expand your experience of a relationship. In addition, it creates karmic attachments to people, places, things, or ideals. Examining the motives underlying a loyalty determines whether the energy attachments are appropriate for spiritual growth. True loyalty is the connection from the Heart with the Soul.

Rosemary oil's energy comforts emotional heartbreak, and is appropriate to use for achieving closure to a relationship. Often when a love is lost suddenly and without closure, a person indulges in a fantasy that the relationship has not ended. Continuously reminiscing on the good memories and denying the reality of why the relationship ended creates an obsessive denial that stunts growth. The root cause of this type of obsession is often insecurity and co-dependency. Rosemary's energy persuades the Self to acknowledge the truth and allow the obsessive behavior to transform into acceptance. It is necessary to learn the lesson that love only generates from within. If you do not love yourself, the need for love will be filled by a substitution that subdues but does not resolve the feelings of loneliness and abandonment felt over the ending of a relationship. Rosemary helps you take responsibility for the relationship by acknowledging how the relationship served you. Learning the lesson allows you to move on.

The grieving process integral to concluding a relationship often affects the lungs. The energetic action of Rosemary promotes the release of grief held in the lungs. On the physical level the oil is good to massage into the chest and lungs for opening up the breath, which nourishes all the organs of the body by increasing the oxygen. Learning to breathe deep into the chest cavity opens heart energy, increasing the ability to feel emotions. Shallow breathing is indicative of people who are more visual and mental. Learning to breathe deeply helps them to become more kinesthetic.

Rosemary's energy helps restore innocence and promotes a return to wholeness. Incest survivors benefit from the oil's soothing and nurturing energy, especially when using it during the recovery process. Energetically, Rosemary transforms incest survivors' feelings of uncleanness and shame, enabling the survivor to recover a sense of self-esteem. The cellular memory of the spleen carries memories of blood ties and incest memories. If these memories remain emotionally traumatic, they may potentially become a disruptive influence on the gallbladder meridian's energy. Embracing the feelings of loyalty and betrayal into love allows the survivor to release some of their self-directed anger and reestablish trust in the survivor's life.

The herb Rosemary helps digest fatty foods. The craving for fatty foods stems from a deep unconscious feeling of not being nourished in life. Often dairy products and chocolate are a substitution for love. Using Rosemary oil helps overcome these cravings.

Using the oil for transformation

Keep Rosemary oil in the medicine chest for its many healing purposes. Rosemary oil works on the physical, emotional, mental, and spiritual levels. Massaging the oil into the gallbladder and spleen meridians accelerates the healing process of an incest survivor. An important point to stimulate for releasing abuse energy is located on the gall bladder meridian at the hip. This will be a very tender point on the exterior side of the hip joint, especially for those carrying memories of abuse in their body. This abuse can be programmed into the cellular memory from this lifetime or others. Do deep massage with Rosemary oil on this area. This promotes release of stagnant energy from the meridian, and over time transforms the feelings of bitterness and resentment. Massaging the oil into the small intestine meridian helps abuse survivors overcome thoughts of being impure and dirty and allows feelings of victimization trapped in the body to begin releasing. Using the oil on the conception meridian reduces feelings of terror and hysteria that a survivor often feels. Massaging oil into the pericardium meridian assists in initiating intimacy. Rubbing the oil on the front and back of the heart and heart meridian increases feelings of self-value and self-worth.

Continued use of Rosemary decreases heart palpitations caused by anxiety. As a massage oil, Rosemary calms the nervous system, and is excellent for cases of nervous itching. Rosemary can alleviate some of the discomfort of shingles. It also helps relieve muscle pain and mild forms of arthritis stiffness by increasing the ability to flow with change. Massaging the large intestine meridian with the oil relaxes obsessive states, and letting go becomes easier.

Headaches in the front of the head are often due to digestive difficulties. Massaging Rosemary on the head and abdomen gives some comfort to these ailments. Hold the point on the webbing between the thumb and first finger to move the energy. Massaging the arms deeply helps release stagnated energy that is instrumental in creating headaches. Drinking a cup of Rosemary herb tea aids digestive ailments and energetically digests new realities and thought forms.

Using Rosemary oil in hair conditioner helps to replenish the pranic energy of the hair and gives it sheen and body. Sheets scented with Rosemary invoke a feeling of security. Put a few drops in the laundry rinse cycle or impregnate a cloth with the oil and put in the dryer.

Precautions

Avoid using during pregnancy. Rosemary oil can be abortive if used internally. If high blood pressure is present, use cautiously in baths and highly diluted as a massage oil, but do not inhale. Rosemary is often diluted with turpentine. This oil is fairly non-irritating, to be certain check for a reaction. Use 15-30 drops in 2 ounces of a base oil.

ROSEWOOD　　　　　　　　　　　*Aniba rosaeodora – Lauraceae*
Transformations

Key: Opens the Inner-Ear and Compassion. Men discover that their inherent feminine qualities are a resource. Women with strong male attributes soften with the energy. Muse-inspired talents are realized; musicians are inspired with heart-generated creativity. Comprehending the power of sound heightens perception and the ability to communicate with different realms.

Growth and healing issues

The porcupine projections and rough edges of the personality smooth with this gentle energy. Feelings of abandonment, loneliness, depression, and sorrow are comforted with the tender and loving nature of Spirit brought by Rosewood. Spiritual attainment cultivates a serene and calm essence that releases emotional pain from grief, loss, or heartbreak. Maintaining the need for protection is a defensive ploy that contributes to emotional detachment and maintains separation. Embracing hurts permits penetration of the armor shielding a person from experiencing pain.

Energetic influences on the bodies and chakras

The tender gentleness of Spirit flows through all the bodies, soothing the pain of separation. The heart energy expands with gentleness and innocence. Creativity heightens when the inner ear opens, expanding the throat, third eye, and heart chakras to actualize Spirit. Calming the energy to flow through all the bodies in continuous balance releases the anxieties that constrict the energy.

Energetics of the oil

The scent of Rosewood is very alluring with a quality that feels faintly familiar and leaves a haunting echo. Rosewood energetically renews acquaintance with one's secret and vulnerable inner essence. It enhances and encourages those energy attributes that reflect the soft and gentle inherent qualities of Spirit, allowing the personality to smooth its rough edges.

Rosewood energy stimulates recognition of undiscovered abilities with a potential for great creativity. The energy of the oil has a unique ability to inspire the unconscious into remembering the forgotten aspects of self, where an abundance of inner resources has accumulated, awaiting realization. It can access talents cultivated in other lifetimes.

Rosewood oil directly influences both the emotional and mental bodies by helping to dissolve internal strife. Energetically, Rosewood dissolves stress by calming the energy. This balances the flow of energy through the physical and subtle bodies, allowing a calm steady energy flow to be felt.

The heart chakra is greatly affected by Rosewood oil's energy. Energetically, it calms feelings of apprehension felt in the heart, allowing the heart to remember what it is like to feel tenderness and contentment. In this way, Rosewood eases feelings of loneliness and abandonment by transforming depression and sadness into feelings of contentment and understanding, which allows for detachment from the past. This does not mean denying or rationalizing feelings, but a resolution to release them by embracing the cause of the inner turmoil. Rosewood aids inner child therapies, especially when feelings and patterns of abandonment developed early in life from the death of a loved one, parental divorce, or the simple lack of a loving environment to nourish the child's heart chakra. A parent's inability to demonstrate heartfelt feelings can leave a child's emotional needs unfulfilled. Later in life that adult child will have difficulty getting their emotional needs met because their role models never demonstrated how. To complicate the situation more, they will have encased themselves in armor to protect their vulnerability. Rosewood oil's energy surfaces the repressed feelings and decisions formed by those early experiences and transforms feelings of abandonment allowing them to realize they do have security in their lives.

Rosewood has a sensuous energy that revives the tender qualities of innocent love, often similar to the feelings of first love. It unleashes the all-encompassing feeling of puppy love that comes without the baggage of past fears, rejection, or hurt. Teenagers going through their first love experience could benefit from Rosewood oil's energy, as it allows them to positively pass through the closure without creating negative attitudes to influence later experiences.

Men respond very favorably to Rosewood oil because it helps them connect into their feminine qualities and promotes engaging their female essence more fully. Rosewood energy feels very nurturing to men. Energetically, Rosewood oil promotes the innate dominating, controlling, logical male energy to harmonize with the gentle, emotionally sensitive, and intuitive female nature. Women with dominating and driven energy also benefit from the softening qualities of this oil.

Rosewood oil's energy brings awareness to unconscious memories of abuse—not being heard or hearing unwanted and detrimental criticism—lodged in the auditory sense. This type of abuse can distort the self-esteem and the ability to be receptive to authority. Listening to verbal abuse severs the connection to inner source and sets up a pattern of needing to be validated by sources outside of self. Self-rebellion begins to calm when using Rosewood oil, and one is receptive to hearing inner Source directives.

Rosewood stimulates hearing the music of the Soul and opens the inner ear to celestial music. Rosewood stimulates creativity in musicians. Rosewood energy is to musicians as Laurel is to artists. Rosewood—the actual wood—is used to make musical instruments. Rosewood energy facilitates the higher abstract mind to align through heart energy. Its energy opens the creativity of the heart and often manifests as latent abilities in music, performing, dance, and poetry.

Deeply inhaling Rosewood oil stimulates the feeling of being in a different world, in a place where the heart inherently knows how to stay open. It is a reality that has a wild and free feeling. It recalls memories of the moon shining into a forest upon a ring of dancing Fairies, Elves, and Gnomes. This is the land of the muse. Energetically, Rosewood strengthens the connection with Nature and Earth Spirits and develops a form of communication with them. Heightening the inner hearing abilities realizes the power of sound. Sound creates form. The reason discordant noise feels abrasive is it produces friction that can misalign the templates between the physical and subtle bodies. Often when a degree of spiritual attainment is achieved, a person begins desiring solitude and cultivates a quiet essence about them. Humanity's noise pollution profoundly effects people, nature, and other dimensions. Rosewood grows only in ancient rainforests, and like the Wood Folk, it is rapidly disappearing.

Using the oil for transformation

Rosewood oil has soothing skin properties and is good for massaging into the neck and face. It is also good for healing scars and wounds and for rejuvenating wrinkles and signs of aging since it addresses the hardening thought patterns of death. Rosewood oil prompts feelings that restore innocence and feeling young again.

Massage Rosewood oil up and down the spine to free the Kundalini energy. Using Rosewood on the front and back of the heart allows a nurturing energy to be felt through all the bodies. Rub on the throat, crown, and third eye chakras to open the center of creative expression and integrate more of the Higher Self into the personality. Massaging the sacral chakra front and back unleashes blocked creativity. Gently massage the oil behind the ears to stimulate inner hearing of etheric sound currents. Rosewood energy also stimulates the pituitary gland, which controls the aging process and reception of the messages from the Higher Mind. Use deep pressure to massage the oil into the pituitary reflex point on either big toe while deeply breathing the oil, to invoke the muses of creativity. To stimulate feelings of being nurtured massage under and on the breasts. Rosewood is a good oil for women that have had breast cancer. Using Rosewood on the triple warmer meridian supports us when facing the unfamiliar aspects of ourselves and bringing them into the light. Massaging the oil behind the ears and into the kidney meridian helps balance and heighten the auditory energy, which supports clearer inner hearing. It provides nourishment to the nervous system, and stimulates the immune system and the thymus chakra.

Precautions

Be suspicious of this oil's purity because it is often diluted with less expensive constituents. This oil is fairly non-irritating, to be certain check for a reaction. Use 15-30 drops in 2 ounces of a base oil.

RUE   *Ruta graveolens – Rutaceae*
Transformations

Key: Illuminates the Truth of Life. Self-esteem is empowered by connecting into inherent wisdom. Increasing self-worth is achieved by embracing Divine Grace. Wisdom through experience embodies Crone energy, and allows one's truth to be realized and spoken.

Growth and healing issues

The personality is freed to welcome Spirit once it transforms the rage, addiction to drama, and other intense passions creating destructive behaviors that maintain separation. Truth illuminates, shattering delusion and denial. Subliminal death wishes are acknowledged. Rue energy addresses persecution and paranoia complexes by stimulating insights into their root-cause.

Energetic influences on the bodies and chakras

Heart energy expands and energy distortions in the lungs release. The root chakra expands to connect with the Earth and promote enthusiasm for living. Rue energy dissipates the disharmonious vibrations that have collected in a room or space.

Energetics of the oil

Rue is known as the "herb of grace," and energetically allows a person to feel worthy of accepting Divine Grace. Rue addresses issues of empowerment and is an antidote for poisoning the self-esteem. Rue can also be poisonous, much as self-esteem is poisonous when it is not motivated from a place of love, but is a defense mechanism directed by fear. Rue's oil is a green color and its energy directly effects the heart and lungs.

Rue illuminates the truth of life. During World War II the Nazis developed a truth serum from Rue. Energetically, Rue shatters the spell of delusion. Ungrounded people with subliminal death wishes can use the energy of Rue to transform that energy into recognition of their existence, which encourages a desire to live. Rue sets the spirit free.

The energy of Rue embodies Scorpio and Mars energy. By releasing angry rage and other intense passions, the oil helps address their destructive behavioral patterns and lets them evolve into more harmonious behaviors. Rue illustrates the intensity of life and is a good oil for drama queens to use, because it absolves the need to create drama by getting to the truth of the matter. Death comes to realities that are no longer conducive to Spiritual evolution. Its energy helps a person realize the things that no longer work in their life, be they thought patterns or beliefs. By releasing these things, the need to experience them again is eliminated. Rue is a beneficial oil to use for introspection into relationships as it dispels illusions, especially relationships based on a dysfunctional fantasy that the collective social conditioning recognizes as truth. Rue energy accelerates closure of inappropriate relationships not built on foundations of love.

There is an old saying, "one who knows uses Rue." It embodies the energy of the Crone, which is the energy of wisdom through experience. Traditionally, Rue guarded against evil spirits and was used to cleanse Pagan temples. Catholic priests used sprigs of Rue to sprinkle holy water. The irony is that Pagans introduced priests to Rue and were later persecuted by the same Christians. Using Rue awakens memories of being persecuted in the Witchhunts. Rue aids in recalling intense memories of lifetimes during the Inquisition, helping overcome the unconscious paranoia and feelings of persecution created by those experiences when that energy bleeds through to the present. People with past life recollections of, or family connections to victims of Nazi concentration camps or other imprisonment would benefit by using Rue. Often those embedded memories keep a person from feeling able to live life openly and aligned with their true spiritual inclinations. This has the potential to generate great internal stress, often making them afraid to voice their opinions for fear they might be noticed—drawing attention brings the possibility of persecution. In spiritual matters, these people might have only a fragile grasp on their beliefs, and this grasp would disintegrate under intense inspection from an authoritarian source. Even without past trauma, people are trained to accept the consensual reality, and this conditioning does not inspire freethinking. When an individual overcomes this programming, but does not have the self-confidence to support their reality, they often begin to feel persecuted for their thoughts. This produces a tendency to be untruthful to Self. Meditating with Rue oil helps resolve these issues by empowering an individual to firmly connect to their own inherent wisdom. Rue is also beneficial for those afraid to own their power.

Using the oil for transformation

Rue is a good oil to use in magical ceremonies or rituals to purify and sanctify a space. Use Rue when laying the foundation for a new home, office, or altar to consecrate the foundation and empower the purpose of the space. It purifies by dissolving dense energy vibrating in a space and channeling in light energies. Rue can be used in a spray or used or warmed in an aromatherapy lamp to clear an environment.

Rue also protects against the energy of psychic attacks. Cleanse a bedroom before going to sleep to protect the space from invading thought forms that produce distressful sleep. Meditate on the issues of persecution and the causes of being emotionally suppressed while inhaling the oil. Use Rue on the conception, triple warmer, and stomach meridians to release obsessions and subliminal death wishes. Using Rue on the kidney meridian helps you become more present and releases fears.

Precautions

The scent is very calming but Rue is too toxic to use undiluted. Do not use as a massage oil because of its toxicity. Ingesting the oil is fatal. Finding pure Rue oil is almost impossible, so you may choose to use the plant for these healings. Never use the oil during pregnancy or on children. Rue oil has a narcotic effect and using too much is dangerous. Rue oil can irritate the skin and mucous membranes. Dilute 1-10 drops in 2 ounces of a base oil. Use only 1-5 drops in a bath.

SAGE (WILD SAGE OR DALMATIAN SAGE)
Salvia officinalis — Labiatae

Transformations

Key: Accesses Ancestral Wisdom. Surrendering to Spirit brings the balance and inner peace that supports standing firm on your path. Feeling nurtured and supported introduces the feeling of a state of Oneness. Trance states are easily induced by dancing and drumming and heighten awareness and perception. Embracing Spirit supports receiving abundance and support.

Growth and healing issues

Knowledge encoded in the DNA activates and filters into the consciousness to manifest. Behaviors of self-judgment, denial, and self-sabotage are recognized. Discovering and using latent resources increases self-sufficiency and overcomes fears and feelings of inadequacy, lack, unfocused direction, and unworthiness.

Energetic influences on the bodies and chakras

Rips and holes in a woman's etheric womb caused by childbirth are repaired. The emotional, mental, physical bodies and aura are purified. Conflicts felt in the digestive system, often caused by resistance to change, begin to resolve. Releasing old beliefs helps overcome resistance by creating a state more receptive to new ideas.

Energetics of the oil

Sage embodies the silver color frequency of illuminating power, imparting the wisdom of our ancestors. Sage energy accesses ancestral knowledge encoded in our DNA. Its energy stimulates reaching inside one's self to realize inherent wisdom. Energetically, Sage unlocks the resources of ancient knowledge.

Traditionally, Native Americans used Sage in purification rituals. Sage encourages people to identify with the Red Road, which instills the harmony of Nature. The Native Americans lived in a state of sacred reverence attuned with the land. Sage strengthens communication with the Unseen Realm. Native Americans traditionally burned Sage. Blowing the smoke around a person's body releases negativity and helps to purify their Spirit. Warming Sage oil in an aromatherapy lamp has the same cleansing effect, releasing mental burden and clearing the environment of emotionally charged vibration.

Sage energy is a mirror for truthfully looking at ourselves. Introspection helps uncover denied issues and self-judgments. Acknowledging and ultimately embracing the energy attached to those issues restores harmony and balance to life. The main issue addressed by Sage oil's energy is self-sabotage. When an aspect of the self undermines growth, a pattern of self destruction develops. The pattern is reinforced by the lack of sufficient resources to flow with change. Sage's energy overcomes self-sabotage patterns by connecting to the wisdom of the elders and bringing the inherent resources necessary for growth. Sage energy helps ease the fear of moving into new situations in life, fortifying the personality's ability to dispel fears and increasing confidence.

The energy of Sage reinforces feelings of independence and resourcefulness. The acceleration of energetic shifts and changes happening in this plane now often lodge as density in the legs. Many people experience aches, pains, and cramps in the legs from this accelerated energy. The legs represent the ability to move forward and resistance to change stagnates energy in the legs. Learning to stand firm on the spiritual path helps surmount these fears. Surrendering to Spirit maintains balance in life and allows issues to resolve in divine right order.

Meditation with Sage oil helps you clearly look at life's essential needs and reveals your expectations of people. It is necessary to examine why another person is required to fill certain needs. Needs indicate that a lack exists in one's self. Learning to be self-sufficient requires attuning to Spirit; anything clsc is a substitution for love and a deficiency of Spirit. Surrendering to Spirit fills lack. It is important to be clear about what your needs are, and maintain focus on your intent to manifest fulfillment. Most of the time the self is not clear about what its needs are, and the intent is focused on what it does not want or what it fears. This intense focus attracts unwanted things to manifest and falls short of providing for true needs. It is very important to be open to receiving what you need. Often the personality feels unworthy and undeserving of receiving what it wants. Using Sage oil for introspection addresses the thought patterns that block the ability to receive and helps develop acceptance.

Sage is a good oil to use when you are not feeling supported in life. Often the personality builds walls for protection. These walls prevent you from feeling nurtured by other people, which magnifies the feeling of not being supported. The walls imprison the self in the state of separation and prevent you from feeling the state of Oneness. Achieving the state of Oneness is the ultimate support in life.

It is important to examine other people's motives to determine if they are supporting or restraining the magnificence of Self that wishes expression. Often, other people feel intimidated by a person with an actualized Self. When they encounter a person with a high degree of actualized Self, those that aren't may exhibit passive aggressive behavior or express hurtful criticism created by their insecurities. When this type of negative personality is present, it is important to do cord cutting for disconnecting their influence.

The energetics of Sage comfort the digestion system. Digestive ailments are often created by resistance to new ideas or by holding onto old, worn-out beliefs. Sage energy facilitates the ability to easily digest change by letting go of old beliefs, thus enabling energy shifts to feel gentler in the physical body.

Sage oil energetically strengthens and repairs the womb energy in women who have birthed children. During pregnancy, a baby's Soul connects through the umbilical cord and moves in and out of this dimensional plane during the gestation of its physical body. The Soul does not completely stay in the physical body until after birth. This process of the Soul bonding with the mother and its new form rips a hole in the mother's etheric womb or aura. Sage helps mend the torn etheric womb. Sage oil also benefits women who have had abortions or miscarriages, because the Soul was moving in and out, deciding whether to stay or not.

Using the oil for transformation

Use Sage oil in meditation to reconnect with ancestral memories. Deeply inhale Sage essence and listen carefully to the ancestral whisperings, restoring forgotten knowledge.

Rubbing Sage oil on the legs releases energy blocked by prolonged standing or poor circulation to the feet. This blocked energy creates the tendency to swell, further hindering the energy flow. Massaging the oil into the stomach and bladder meridian rejuvenates the legs and releases the stagnated energy creating tiredness. Shaking the legs helps to move blocked energy. A massage therapist or body worker can use Sage oil for a spinal clearing, which promotes a balanced energy flow. This is done by massaging the oil on the spine and holding one hand at the sacrum while the other hand moves the energy up the spine to clear energetic blocks. When the hand reaches base of the skull, send energy up and down the spine between the hands, to energize the person receiving the treatment. Rocking the body helps release blockages.

Massaging Sage oil into the bladder meridian alleviates back pain, promoting feelings of support and inducing an openness to receiving. Sage oil can be helpful in relieving sciatic nerve pain (the nerve that starts at the hip and runs down the outside of the leg to the foot). Using Sage oil on the gallbladder meridian relieves sciatica and lower back pain. Rubbing the oil on the lung and large intestine meridians will help open the ability to "let go and let come" which furthers acceptance of self. To promote self-nurturing, massage the oil into the stomach meridian. To repair the etheric womb, focus intention while massaging Sage oil into the abdominal region as well as the conception, spleen, and liver meridians.

Precautions

Do not use this oil on children or infants. Avoid using during pregnancy. If you have epilepsy, be careful inhaling and using externally. If high blood pressure is present, use cautiously in baths and highly diluted as a massage oil, but do not inhale. This oil can be slightly irritating to the skin and potentially sensitizing; check for a reaction. Dilute 15-20 drops of oil in 2 ounces of base oil.

SANDALWOOD   *Santalum album – Sanlalacea*
Transformations

Key: Awakens Divine Sensuality. Multi-sensory abilities heighten which helps to perceive subtle energy emanations. This expansion allows greater reception of intuitive messages from Source. The imagination is stimulated, permitting it to perceive, receive, and experience the gift of Spiritual abundance.

Growth and healing issues

Sexual passions calm into the state of Divine sacredness. Uniting root chakra energy with the heart brings calm and grounds the Kundalini energy into the physical. Motivations of sexual urges are realized, allowing the experience of true love. Recognizing that feeling is more than pain stimulates a desire to truly feel. Strengthening the emotional body's bond with the physical generates greater satisfaction and allows one to become more present and conscious in the physical body.

Energetic influences on the bodies and chakras

Energy distortions in the root and sacral chakras release once embraced and aligned with the heart energy. Expanding root and sacral chakra energy encourages a more Divine experience of sexuality. Stimulating the Kundalini helps transform karma that is distorting the energy in each of the chakras.

Energetics of the oil

Sandalwood's scent invokes a feeling of exotic sensuality and calmness. Spirit evolves by awakening the Kundalini and quieting the sexual energies. Energetically, Sandalwood aligns and balances the heart with the sacral chakra's feminine energies and the root chakra's male energies.

This alignment liberates the stored Kundalini energy coiled in the base of the spine. Releasing this energy grounds and connects the energy to the heart. Sandalwood calms sexual urges and brings them into a state of wholeness, facilitating learning the true sense of love. Additional exploration into the nature of true love brings forth comprehension of the sexual nature's Divine sacredness.

Sandalwood awakens true sensuality and full perception through all the senses. Prolonged use of Sandalwood with meditation to focus the intention teaches you to use all the senses to feel. This awareness requires that you be totally in your body and learn to feel all the subtle energy around you. Feeling becomes more than an awareness of pain caused by injuring the ego.

Sandalwood has been used through the centuries as a meditation incense. It brings calmness and promotes a greater contentment with Self. This calms allows reception of intuitive messages from Source. The imagination is stimulated and the mental body's control loosens, allowing the personality to experience the abundance of Spirit. Using Sandalwood initiates feelings that anything is possible.

Sandalwood oil is produced in the heartwood of the tree. The Sandalwood tree is native to Asia. Ancient Sanskrit and Chinese writings describe many uses of Sandalwood. It has a rich tradition of religious uses and many divine images and temple relics were carved from the wood. The Egyptians imported it for their religious purposes. The Indian Ayurvedic system uses it for many therapeutic applications. Sandalwood awakens past-life experiences and memories of many cultures, which is why the scent feels and smells so familiar.

Using the oil for transformation

Rubbing Sandalwood on the sacrum area and up the spine and neck produces a wonderful feeling. Massage the oil into the belly and pubic bone for opening the sacral and root chakras. To feel sensual, rub Sandalwood oil on the inner wrists, behind the ears, and on the chest.

The bronchial tubes and chest respond favorably to the oil. Sandalwood can energetically open the lungs when rubbed on the back lung area and lung reflex points on both the hands and feet. After rubbing on the body, do deep breathing to achieve deeper states of relaxation. Massage along the bladder meridian to release suppressed feelings of sexuality and increase virility. Using on the small intestine meridian to help separate pure from impure thoughts and helps overcome sexual complexes. Massaging the pericardium meridian with the oil allows intimacy to be felt. Using on the liver meridian helps overcome frigidity.

Precautions

Be suspicious of this oil's purity because it is often diluted with synthetics or less expensive constituents. This oil is fairly non-irritating, to be certain check for a reaction. Use 15-30 drops in 2 ounces of a base oil.

SASSAFRAS   *Sassafras albidum – Lauraceae*

Transformations

Key: Heightens Discernment. Releasing judgments raises the vibrational rate and provides an environment that supports a state of allowance. Greater flexibility and spontaneity allow the feeling of profound joy. Discerning between the needs for Spiritual growth and ego desires brings abundance. Spiritual guidance transforms the rigid convictions of mass consciousness. Learning to wisely use power aligned with Spirit begins by disconnecting from the ego's power.

Growth and healing issues

Understanding the root causes of feelings of rage, frustration, willful ego, and pride confirm that they are unnecessary defensive reactions which do not protect but harm. Understanding the difference between control and responsibility is realized through allowance and acceptance. Learning the correct use of power promotes Spiritual growth. Taking responsibility for actions promotes making conscious choices. Divine surrender and acceptance reduce resistance to change and support making choices instead of reactions.

Energetic influences on the bodies and chakras

Clearing the solar plexus chakra energetically balances the emotions and overcomes the tendencies of control and manipulation. Aligning the third eye, heart, and solar plexus energies helps Spiritual purpose direct the will. The vibration rate increases by coming into alignment with Spiritual purpose.

Energetics of the oil

Sassafras is like the feeling of being in an old musty barn; it piques the curiosity to search for hidden treasure—the treasures of Self. Sassafras is a powerful oil for clearing and stimulating the solar plexus energy. The energetics of Sassafras stimulate the emotional courage to increase feelings of self-love.

Feelings that originate from the center of ego—gut feelings—are most active and open in the mass consciousness. Often these gut emotions are the only emotions a person is able to feel. These are the emotions of hurt pride and ego concerns. The solar plexus's denser energies are based on insecurity, control, and manipulation that arise from the old reality of competition-based survival. Sassafras energy helps overcome the rigid convictions of the mass consciousness by uniting the energies of the solar plexus with the heart. Energetically, Sassafras oil balances the emotions by supplying the energy to examine convictions and determine if they create limitations and obstacles that hinder spiritual growth. It creates an opportunity to comprehend the lessons and experiences of power and ego and culminates in learning how to wisely use power and the ego to promote spiritual growth.

Sassafras generates the ability to take responsibility for manifesting your life situations and experiences by balancing and aligning the heart energy with the raw gut feelings of the solar plexus chakra. It supports understanding how the right use of will shapes and manifests reality and how every situation in life is an opportunity to spiritually grow. Connecting the solar plexus/ego-will center with the heart empowers the alignment of energy with Spiritual purpose. It is important to keep conscious intention directed on training and firmly establishing this alignment. Falling back to the reality of ego manipulation happens naturally just by being human. It is necessary to constantly focus our intent to be heart conscious. Sassafras oil energetically raises the solar plexus energy up into the heart so that it can expand and evolve into a more spiritual-based energy.

Sassafras aligns the solar plexus and third eye chakras for greater intuitive awareness. Opening the third eye with an aligned solar plexus harmonizes the energy of will with spiritual sight. Outer awareness shifts to the inner realm of true Source. To stay connected with Source, the emotional body needs to release feelings of rage, anger, frustration, willful ego, and pride. Those feelings keep personal power and spiritual purposes in denial. Not taking one's power keeps the energy field in a state of density and vibrating at a lower frequency. Not taking power keeps the interpretation of life on an ego based level.

Sassafras oil can be used to explore issues contributing to the lack of abundance. Sassafras helps raise an understanding about what desiring something means. The inner self interprets desire as an existence of a state of lack. Spiritual truth declares that only abundance exists. The energetics of Sassafras oil helps learning to discern between ego desires and Spiritual direction, and promotes the understanding that anything is possible and within reach. It supports feeling that the self is worthy to receive the abundance of Spirit.

The Sassafras tree is native to North America, and the Iroquois people of the eastern United States honored the tree as sacred because it provided them with many healing remedies. The sixteenth-century Spaniards took cuttings and the knowledge of its therapeutic uses back to Spain. Sassafras awakens memories of the collective consciousness of Native American life times and of sixteenth-century explorers of the New World.

Using the oil for transformation

Massaging Sassafras into the sacral and solar plexus chakras helps to open and align both of them. Massage the oil into the pancreas area to balance the etheric hormones throughout the body. Creating more laughter in life helps align all the chakras with Spirit. Use the oil on the stomach meridian to encourage feelings of self-acceptance. Sassafras on the liver meridian harmonizes and integrates self and develops the ability to take full responsibility for actions. Massage above the knees to stimulate the release of heart hormones.

Precautions

This essential oil can be internally toxic and potentially lethal. Avoid using during pregnancy. Do not use this oil on children or infants. This oil can irritate the skin and mucous membranes. Dilute 1-10 drops in 2 ounces of a base oil. Use only 1-5 drops in a bath.

SAVORY
Satureja hortensis (summer) / Satureja montana (winter) – Labiatae
Transformations

Key: Overcomes Domination and Control. Attuning to the Animal Kingdom enhances and strengthens the bond with Earth. This allows Humanity to experience unconditional love and the joy of living in the moment. Allowance transforms rigid beliefs that maintain separation.

Growth and healing issues

Surrendering the ego's need to be in control leads to experiencing the state of Oneness. A secure foundation of Spiritual self-love stimulates a desire for intimacy and awakens dormant sexual energy. Spiritual energy inspires healthier attitudes about intimacy. Root causes contributing to sexual problems are revealed and healing begins, allowing a richer experience of sexual pleasures. The powerful influence of sexual projections is realized and more appropriate uses of the energy can be utilized.

Energetic influences on the bodies and chakras

Aligning the heart and solar plexus chakras begins moving the dense gut energy through the heart to transform it. Ego wounds that build walls and defenses diminish with self-love and understanding of their harmful influence on the personality and Spiritual growth. Savory energy eases the emotional hurts that distort the root and sacral chakras' energy.

Energetics of the oil

Savory implies desire and illuminates the animalistic nature of Humanity. Meditating with Savory oil summons the satyr Pan, half man and half beast. Savory energy helps you recognize the internal beast. "Civilized" man has denied this aspect of self, resulting in a fragmented self filled with frustration and anger.

Energetically, Savory addresses the need to dominate and control. Savory energy imparts understanding of insecurities and relinquishes the need to control and to be superior. Separation from Source contributes to promoting domination and manipulation. The personality learns lessons from experiences of manipulation and forms a desire to temper Spirit with allowance. Allowance transforms rigid and limiting beliefs, enabling a greater understanding of abundance. Divine surrender to the God-Self resolves any need for control. Once the state of Oneness is achieved it will eliminate the need for control and manipulation. Furthermore, once Humanity achieves the understanding and experience of Oneness, it will fulfill its rightful destiny as true co-creators in the Garden of Eden.

Savory works on the mental plane, energetically soothing feelings of emotional hurt. Emotional injury can be caused by other people's harmful thought projections. Also, when the ego feels wounded, it often directs detrimental energy inwards towards the self. Savory's energy releases frustrations and sustains a more loving state.

Historically, Savory was used as an aphrodisiac to encourage lusty animal nature. Its energy awakens the sexual nature. Sex energy is a connection of the root and sacral chakras. When sexual energy moves up into the heart, it becomes love. This deep bond inspires a spiritual way to lovingly share one's self with another human.

Energetically, Savory accesses the root causes of sexual problems. Introspection while using Savory will help recover the deep-rooted causes of frigidity or impotence. Sometimes the cause stems from shame or guilt, frequently from religious teachings that sex is bad. Sexual issues can generate from past lives of debauchery or abstinence.

Also, intense fantasies or sexual lust projected at another person can pervert sexual energy and can be damaging to the person who is the object of this projection. It can be a subtle feeling, or it can generate feelings of being attacked. If this energy is projected constantly over time, the person receiving this energy begins to feel it is unsafe to initiate intimacy. If the person is very sensitive, it will feel like being raped. Such is the case of a father lusting after his daughter: the daughter unconsciously perceives this energy from her father, and it has a potential to create distorted relationship models that will affect her future relationships. Massage therapists often experience this phenomenon: they feel uneasy or physically uncomfortable while working on certain male clients. Often the client is relaxing and opening to emotion the only way he knows, which is sexually. To be truly responsible for your actions, be aware of how powerful the mental body's projections are. Using Savory to align the energy of the root and sacral chakras and bond the energy with the heart immediately transforms sexual energy distortions and allows a person to experience fulfilling ecstasy.

Savory energy helps us attune to and communicate with the Animal Kingdom, and recognize that we humans have an animal nature. Animals have much to teach those who listen because they know unconditional love and the joy of being in the moment. Savory renews our connection to Earth energy and stimulates archetypal Goddess energy, reinforcing our bond with Gaia. Savory reminds us to treat Her with the sacred reverence she deserves. Restoring our bond with nature ensures true harmony will influence our lives. Summer Savory has an affinity with the summer solstice and the solstice is an excellent time to use the oil, as it ushers in the golden energy of wisdom that enlightens the Soul.

Using the oil for transformation

When the aura is torn, Savory sprayed around the body energetically renews the luminous egg containing an individual's energy field. Savory heals scars on the physical body caused by burns, cuts, bites, and boils, and alleviates mouth ulcers, all symbols of anger directed inwards. It also works on acne, another manifestation of self-disgust.

Warming Savory in an aromatherapy lamp clears the environment of discordant energy, allowing healing harmony to perpetuate. Savory can work on the etheric level to assimilate vitamins and minerals for manifesting a strong physical form. It also works on the physical to stop bleeding. Use on the pericardium and heart meridians and the root and sacral chakras to release sexual blockages.

Precautions

Do not use this oil on children or infants. Avoid using during pregnancy. This oil can irritate the skin and mucous membranes. Dilute 1-10 drops in 2 ounces of a base oil and check for a reaction. Use only 1-5 drops in a bath.

SPEARMINT   *Mentha spicata– Labiatae*

Transformations

Key: Ionizes the Etheric Body. Establishing boundaries and taking responsibility for one's truth develops integrity and diminishes feelings of self-hatred and self-disgust.

Growth and healing issues

Greater self-trust allows feeling protected and safe enough to become vulnerable. More joy and love are felt when the mental body releases the worries that keep it fatigued and drained. Walls and barriers are recognized as defenses maintaining the state of separation.

Energetic influences on the bodies and chakras

Energetically ionizing the etheric body rejuvenates the physical body. The blocked emotions held in the region between the solar plexus and heart chakras are released when they are embraced. Spearmint's refreshing and rejuvenating energy cleanses the emotional and mental bodies.

Energetics of the oil

Spearmint energy feels similar to taking a breath of revitalizing spring air after a cleansing rain. It energetically ionizes the etheric body. This oil rejuvenates energy by cleansing the emotional and mental bodies. Mental fatigue lifts, making it easier to feel comfortable and balanced, while enabling states of love and joy to be more readily felt.

Blocked emotions held in the region between the solar plexus and heart chakra are released by Spearmint oil's energy. Emotions become stuck in that region because of the walls we create for protection from the pain of vulnerability. These walls only create an illusion of protection. In truth, walls create separation and denial of feelings and require a great amount of energy to build and maintain.

Energetically, Spearmint helps assimilate and digest feelings about Self by establishing integrity. Learning to say no and making boundaries for your truth builds integrity. Taking responsibility for your actions and decisions reinforces your truth. Being true to your feelings results in overcoming anger and self-hatred, while restoring self-trust.

Using the oil for transformation

Spearmint massaged on the abdomen and rib cage helps release feelings of self-disgust. Applying pressure to the point approximately one inch below the sternum or the breastbone helps open the breath of life.

Massaging and applying pressure to tender points on the front of the 5th and 6th ribs stimulates hormones going to the heart. The point in the soft tissue above the middle of the kneecap also regulates heart hormones. Dabbing Spearmint oil on the temples creates an uplifting feeling. Use as a spray to ionize a room and the aura.

Precautions

This oil is fairly non-irritating, to be certain check for a reaction. Use 15-30 drops in 2 ounces of a base oil. Spearmint oil reduces the effectiveness of homeopathic remedies.

TANGERINE (MANDARIN)   *Citrus reticulata - Rutaceae*
Transformations

Key: Consciously Present and Aware. Recognizing that change promotes growth enables you to diminish resistance to it. Change can be realized without catastrophe or chaos once the resistance is released. Having faith to create what you need in life helps you live apart from the reality of mass consciousness. New directions and goals feel obtainable.

Growth and healing issues

Embracing change with enthusiasm and joy stimulates and enhances the life force. Understanding dawns that change can generate the courage to truly appreciate the gift of life. Spiritual energy assimilates into the personality and motivates its actions. Having the courage to believe and actualize your unique reality keeps you true to your Soul and opens you to infinite possibilities and choices. Victims and enablers in recovery are encouraged to take control of their lives.

Energetic influences on the bodies and chakras

The nervous system calms, which promotes protection while in the dream state. Greater self-expression is actualized as the energies of the root, sacral, and solar plexus chakras align with the throat chakra. Unifying these aligned energies with the third eye produces visions of new possibilities. The cellular memory releases old programming, allowing easier acceptance of new paradigms.

Energetics of the oil

The scent of Tangerine promotes a desire to be more consciously present. Tangerine brings an inherently delightful life force to enhance the energies of the physical, emotional, and mental bodies. It energetically stimulates the ability to look at change with enthusiasm and joy instead of dread and fear. It sparks greater receptivity, letting you accept the gifts life has to offer.

Energetically, Tangerine helps you realize life's sparkle. Children are attracted to its scent of youthful, innocent energy. Tangerine energy can help a repressed inner child to feel and experience joy again. It generates the courage the inner child needs to befriend the adult self. The energy anchors a sunny disposition and stimulates the mental body to perceive the brighter side of life, helping to overcome pessimism and fear. Use Tangerine oil when feeling irritable—its orange color embodies the frequency of courage and optimism and stimulates sociability. It benefits shy people by enabling easier social interaction with strangers and also increasing comfort in new situations. Tangerine energy is excellent to use when networking or speaking in public because it promotes calm when meeting and talking with strangers. Tangerine energy calms nervous tension, very beneficial when experiencing a disturbance in sleep patterns. It also allows the creativity of the dream state to be interpreted by the conscious mind.

Tangerine oil expands abilities to acquire information from Source. It helps manifest the energy of Higher Mind's abstract thought as tangible applications in the physical realm. It supports the formulation of new ideas and beliefs often contrary to the old realities prevalent in society. Tangerine oil's energy stimulates the courage to believe in your self and energetically facilitates disengagement from mass consciousness. Conservative people, those caught up in the complacency of security and comfort that leads them to avoid change benefit from using this oil. Often complacent people live in a reality dependent on a steady paycheck to keep up their standard of living; their apathy to change seduces them into slavery. To most people the thought of making change creates more pain than actual change. When they embark on self-discovery, they often attract intense situations that upset the status quo in their lives. They create this reality by their belief that pain is necessary to make change, alas, "no pain, no gain." They live in the mass reality, unaware that change will set them free. This tendency has the potential to either keep them spiritually impoverished or produce astonishing spiritual growth. The energetics of Tangerine oil lends the courage to make change comfortably, without the traumatic drama. When you learn to create your own reality, you will find that you want to live there. Disconnecting from the collective consciousness raises fears of whether you can survive. Energetically Tangerine lets you feel the resources you have to draw upon for creating your path and walking it.

The energy of the oil aligns the root, sacral, and solar plexus chakras with the throat chakra for articulating greater self-expression. This unified energy stimulates greater creativity when aligned with the third eye energy and lets new possibilities be conceived. This alignment stimulates a greater amount of energy coming into the crown to flow unimpeded through the physical and emotional bodies. Spiritual energy is integrating into the personality. Once the energy flows unimpeded into consciousness, it is easier to manifest new realities, resulting in feelings of success and fulfillment.

Aligning the lower chakras surfaces many issues that have suppressed self-expression. Tangerine is a good oil for people recovering from the role patterns of being a victim or a care-taker, as it fortifies their spirit for learning to live life on their own terms. Tangerine also helps people coming out of relationships to feel receptive of the support and nurturing provided by their Spiritual essence. Tangerine oil's energy helps alleviate the stress created by transiting through these changes. Energetically, Tangerine oil calms the nervous system, and is very beneficial when going through energy shifts, as it supports easier assimilation of the new energy. This calmness of energy promotes discovering your dreams by establishing feelings of wellbeing and joyfulness and awakening inner resources of courage. Use Tangerine oil for marriages, births, or when embarking on new life paths because it stimulates optimism. Use it for celebrating new beginnings, starting new projects, or life changes. Spray Tangerine in the birthing room—it clears and opens the energy so the newborn feels calm and comforted in its new environment.

Brides traditionally walked on a path strewn with the flowers of Mandarin trees, because it was believed to promote fertility. Tangerine energy brings memories of lifetimes in the Orient and Middle East.

Using the oil for transformation

Anoint head points to release the crown and third eye energy. Tangerine is wonderful to use on the spine to unleash Kundalini energy. On the kidney meridians, Tangerine helps overcome any fears of moving into new situations. Tangerine is a good massage oil for releasing edema or stagnated water in the body. Massage on the ankles, hands, and fingers if retaining water. This stimulates the stagnant energy to move out of the body. Massaging the oil behind the knees helps release collected inertia that leads to procrastination and on the solar plexus to strengthen intention. Warming the oil feels very exotic and stimulates a refreshing feeling. It feels good to put a dab on the inner wrist and behind the ears.

Use on the conception meridian to overcome any birth terror and on the governing meridian to releasing constrictions and overcome terror. Spray the oil to dispel any negativity or charged emotions in the environment. It enhances the absorption of Prana into the physical body. Tangerine helps attract abundance of money and success into life and internally promotes feelings of prosperity. Aligning the solar plexus with the etheric body's template allows a steady interchange of energy—it also alleviates hiccups. Hiccups are symptomatic of misaligned energy.

Close your eyes and inhale the oil and allow yourself to travel with the energy to those faraway places where creativity dwells outside the physical realm.

Precautions

Be suspicious of this oil's purity because it is often diluted with synthetics or less expensive constituents. Citrus oils often have a high concentration of pesticides. Keep exposure to sunlight at a minimum when using this oil because this oil can be photosensitizing. This oil can be slightly irritating to the skin and potentially sensitizing; check for a reaction. Diluted15-20 drops of oil in 2 ounces of base oil.

TARRAGON   *Artemisia dracunculus—Asteraceae*
Transformations

Key: An Energetic Shock Rescue Remedy. Provides energy for addressing crises and embracing them as choices made to stimulate change. Shattered fragments of the self are reunited into a state of wholeness and the defensive triggers that close the heart are recognized. Spiritual enthusiasm radiates through the personality's gloom.

Growth and healing issues

Tarragon energy overcomes the shock of a sudden disconnection from Source energy instigated by startling fright or mental or emotional breakdowns. Overcomes traumatic situations that shatter the peace in life or leave you feeling fragile. When the heart energy is constricted or closed it stimulates the need to fill the void with substitutions for love.

Energetic influences on the bodies and chakras

Awakens the life-force within the body. It acts as an energetic shield to diffuse the force of Spiritual impact upon the nervous system, assuring the physical body does not become over stimulated by too much Spiritual energy. The scent grounds one into the physical body by pulling the energy down into the first chakra, opening a feeling of greater stability and connection with Earth energy.

Energetics of the oil

The aroma of Tarragon is very startling. The oil awakens the life force within the body. It is an energetic rescue remedy for treating states of shock caused by a sudden fright or mental or emotional break-downs. Shock occurs when the heart suddenly closes, resulting in a quick constriction of energy that obstructs the flow of light and love that nourishes the physical body.

Energetically Tarragon creates a physical shield, diffusing the force of Spiritual impact upon the nervous system and assuring that the physical body is not over-stimulated by too much Spiritual energy. It acts much like a voltage regulator. It has a calming influence on the mental body, making it possible to overcome confusion. Tarragon oil lets spiritual enthusiasm radiate through the personality's gloom, creating a ray of hope shining light onto the path of new beginnings. Tarragon is useful during a healing crisis to generate the energy necessary to embrace issues.

Tarragon energy shields the solar plexus chakra from the bombardment of external influences. This bombardment feels similar to an attack and can be overwhelming. Resistance to energy causes great discomfort and confusion in the physical body and can upset the digestive system, creating symptoms of gas, ulcers, heartburn. The scent of Tarragon grounds the body by pulling the energy down into the first chakra, opening a greater sense of stability and connection with Earth energy.

Tarragon has a tremendous ability to reunite fragments of self into the whole. Energetically it glues the shattered fragments together. Tarragon is an excellent oil to use during traumatic situations that shatter the peace in life—illness, divorce, unemployment, or just being at a crossroad. Tarragon keeps the heart open during dark periods, letting you see through the shadows to where other possibilities are waiting. Manifesting their possibility only requires placing your focus upon them. Tarragon oil provides the energy to address crises and embrace them as a choice you made to stimulate change, which lets transformation begin to actualize.

Using the oil for transformation

Energetically, Tarragon oil brings a person out of shock by startling them into the present, disengaging their attention from fear. Tarragon is a shock absorber or an emotional rescue remedy when a big realization comes into awareness. It is especially good to use when a big "AH HA!" knocks you backward, over-whelming you with the realization of how long you labored under a false assumption. Truth can be a shock to the system. Great resistance to the truth can rip a hole in the aura, tearing an entrance for truth to come into awareness. Inhale the scent of Tarragon and rub the oil on your hands, then pass your hands around the outside of the luminous egg, or aura. This repairs any tears and gen-erates more energy flow through the etheric body. Tarragon oil's energy will realign all the subtle bodies with the physical. It is a great oil to use during regression or hypnotherapy to recall traumatic experiences, keeping the heart open so the energy attached to a traumatic memory does not close it. Another attribute of Tarragon oil's jolting energy supports staying present. Maintaining focus promotes the choice not to reenact the response patterns that a memo-ry might provoke. Use the oil on the heart region and the heart and pericardi-um meridians to open and balance the energy. Use on the conception meridi-an to overcome terror, and on the kidney meridian to overcome fears.

Precautions

This oil can irritate the skin and mucous membranes. Dilute 1-10 drops in 2 ounces of a base oil and check for a reaction. Use only 1-5 drops in a bath. Avoid using during pregnancy. Do not use this oil on children or infants.

TEA TREE   *Melaleuca alternifolia – Myrtaceae*
Transformations

Key: Reflects the Soul Energy. The shadow self begins to transform into the radiant body. The light body is firmly anchored into the physical body.

Growth and healing issues

New consciousness is inspired as the density of the shadow self is recog-nized. Mental stress and emotional hurts begin to ease and discharge when new perspectives are realized. The ability to change becomes easier as the toxic effects of resistance are released from cellular memory. The internal stress generated by sexual conflict and learned behaviors begins resolving when new insights and attitudes are acquired about sexuality and sexually transmitted disease.

Energetic influences on the bodies and chakras

Tea Tree energy expands all the chakras and aligns them with the crown, establishing new beliefs and social norms. A soothing energy overcomes mental stress and thoughts maintaining the reality of separation. The light body expands, reflecting the radiance of Soul in contrast to the shadow self with its density of fears.

Energetics of the oil

Tea Tree has an intriguing scent—initially it reeks of turpentine, then an undertone of sweetness arises. The scent changes with increased use and when issues transform. Tea Tree is ambrosia to Spirituality.

Tea Tree addresses the victim mentality of the Piscean Age of suffering and guilt. It relinquishes the energy of the Piscean Age's martyr role, and ushers in the Aquarium Age's Grace. Tea Tree energy represents the New Age. It is a new oil, unencumbered with crystallized archetypal energy. It embodies the element of air, facilitating spiritual breath. Tea Tree originates in Australia, which is the heart chakra of the Earth (America is the crown chakra). Therefore, Tea Tree energy expands the heart chakra and etheric lungs.

Energetically, Tea Tree works with the reflection of the Soul as opposed to the shadow self. It expands the energy outwards, reflecting the light body. The light body is the reflection of the radiance of Soul light, while the shadow self is created from fears and rigid consciousness. Tea Tree's energy helps to transform the shadow self into the radiant body, enabling the Shining Self to project. This quality makes Tea Tree instrumental for anchoring the light body to manifest into the physical plane. Tea Tree oil's energy provides great future possibilities. It facilitates the opening of hundreds of dormant chakras, inactive because of the density maintained in the physical body.

Tea Tree oil has a very invigorating energy which releases mental stress and soothes shattered emotional feelings. Once trauma and stress release from the consciousness, old thought patterns can be replaced with new attitudes and energies. Energetically, Tea Tree oil transforms resistance into the ability to change easily. This engages cellular regeneration of the physical and etheric bodies. When cells regenerate, old destructive thought patterns are not reprogrammed into them. The heart chakra and mental body realize the detrimental thought patterns that support the state of separation. Living in a state of divine acceptance and allowance is enabled. The third eye chakra expands, generating new awareness. Tea Tree oil expands all the chakras and aligns them with crown chakra energy for establishing new paradigms.

The Tea Tree grows in dense thickets and dangerous areas of the wild, where poisonous snakes, spiders, and plants grow and thrive. Tea Tree energy lives within a toxic environment but is not affected by it. Similarly, Tea Tree oil engages the body's immune system, stimulating the ability to ward off toxic effects be they emotional, mental, or physical. Tea Tree also has important anti-bacteria and anti-fungal attributes. When the body stays in a prolonged state of agitation or lacks joy, it opens an opportunity for the invasion of bacterial and viral infections. Using the oil in soaps and bath lotions helps enact a barrier of protection for the physical body. It is beneficial for healing any rips or openings in the outer etheric egg.

On the physical level, the oil provides a healing relief for yeast conditions and candida. This condition results from not trusting in relationships, including the relationship with self. Systemic candida infections are caused by prolonged periods of emotional and mental confusion, frustration, and agitation. Eating sugar or using antibiotics establishes an environment for yeast to thrive. Tea Tree gives relief to herpes pains. Herpes conditions result from guilt and shame due to not expressing and validating one's self. This creates bitterness and resentment in the mental body. Another root cause of herpes is conflicting sexual beliefs creating dissonance between internal beliefs and social conditioning—what is the proper and "good" attitude defined by society versus what a person feels to be their truth. This conflict often maintains feelings of shame.

Apprehension over AIDS is distorting the energy of sexuality, creating unhealthy fears. AIDS often terrifies people away from developing loving relationships, promoting mental sex (like phone sex) which inhibits important human contact. Tea Tree energy addresses issues pertaining to sexual shame, energetically reducing religious guilt over sexual issues. Not resolving the conflict of these issues depresses the immune system, opening the opportunity for a virus to run rampant within the body. Confusion defeats the body's ability to fight off viruses.

Using the oil for transformation

Tea Tree oil energetically supports overcoming the programming to have children and the guilt for not. Use Tea Tree in combination with Celery and Carrot Seed oils to facilitate resolving the conflict created by social conditioning to be a parent and helps make the decision whether or not to have children.

Tea Tree oil is instrumental to clearing the energetic field. Tea Tree is a good antiseptic to spray in environments that breed germs. The oil purifies the poisons or pus around a wound and accelerates its healing. The energy regenerates burned skin tissue. Burns stem from festering anger needing release. Tea Tree alleviates the annoyance of athlete's foot symptoms, a condition that energetically results from feelings of non-acceptance and running away from self. Tea Tree also helps gum disease heal, a condition that also indicates suppressed anger.

Massaging on the heart and pericardium meridians releases crystallized emotions, those maintaining a closed heart. Massage above the knee to release heart hormones. Mediation with the oil is very uplifting and expanding, restoring the spirit of delight, which transmutes the dark shadow into the light. Energetically, it regenerates the Soul's connection with the personality, which is the fountain of youth. It was not the right time for

Ponce de Leon to find the fountain, but now with the expansion of consciousness, it is possible.

Precautions

This oil is fairly non-irritating, to be certain check for a reaction. Use 15-30 drops in 2 ounces of a base oil.

VANILLA   *Vanilla planifolia – Orchidaceae*

Transformations

Key: Spiritualizes the Sense of Taste. The light body is refined. Opening to the Higher Mind allows abstract thought to be interpreted and manifested into the physical.

Growth and healing issues

Assists during transitional periods when only light is needed for sustenance. The physical body feels nurtured and not denied while it is adjusting to receiving nourishment totally from light. The palate is purified and fine-tuned and the taste buds to become light receptors. The throat chakra takes on the digestive system's function of metabolizing energy.

Energetic influences on the bodies and chakras

The mental body comes into alignment with the throat, heart, and crown chakras, allowing self-expression to be motivated by love.

Energetics of the oil

The scent of Vanilla brings to mind cookies baking, which recalls warm nurturing memories of a special treat. Energetically, Vanilla spiritualizes the sense of taste.

The energetics of Vanilla clear the palate from craving the taste of physical food. When the light body expands and fully integrates with the physical, nourishment may be received through light. Vanilla purifies the palate and fine-tunes the taste buds for receiving light frequencies. With light body expansion, it will be unnecessary to eat food. The energy creates the production of new amino acids in the brain, and the increased inner light will employ them.

Nourishing energy will be received through the throat chakra. The body will begin digesting the air (or light, so to speak). Vanilla will open the throat's ability to metabolize light, performing the digestive system's function. Through the throat's increasing ability to metabolize light, and the need to eat food will decrease. Using Vanilla can ease and enhance this transitional period. People often crave foods containing Vanilla, which is common in sugary products. Be aware that it is Vanilla being craved not the sweets. Inhaling Vanilla oil accesses the memory of physical food, helping the body to feel nourished in a traditional way. Using Vanilla in this way does not deny the body of any pleasure and reduces its craving for food. It will become a transitional crutch to use before shifting into this new reality, promoting the body to change its relationship with food.

Awakening the etheric palate allows the experience of tasting light and lead to heightened sensitivity. Consequently, you develop the ability to taste whatever is rubbed into the skin. This will change the type of products you use to those based on natural ingredients. An intolerance to using lotions or bug sprays because of their toxic nature might form. Air quality becomes important. Polluted air creates a tendency for developing rashes and allergies in the physical body. This heightened sensitivity may possibly encourage a lifestyle or location change to reduce trauma until the body learns to adjust to this expansion in taste and transmute environmental toxins.

Vanilla invokes turquoise energy, which expands the power center of self-expression by aligning the yellow of the mental body with the green of the heart chakra and the blue of the throat chakra. The mixture of these colors creates turquoise, which harmonizes with the heart chakra, allowing a deeper emotional connection with life. It opens the Higher Mind's ability to feel emotions and execute easier and faster manifestations. The throat chakra automatically opens to the higher energy frequency of the abstract thought of the Higher Mind. Vanilla oil's energy facilitates interpreting the abstract and expressing it in words through a heightened perception of symbolic energy and form. It helps the abstract manifest into form through artistic endeavor, or allows ideas to be articulated.

The Vanilla bean represents the fruition of labor. It is a very condensed energy and symbolically depicts the kernel of truth in a person. It represents the seed of an individual's intent awaiting germination and manifestation. In a fertile mind, abstract consciousness facilitates unlimited physical manifestations. Vanilla is an excellent oil for people working in the metaphysical, philosophical, or scientific fields because it promotes the ability to interpret and express abstract thought in a manner that the masses can comprehend. Vanilla's energy benefits teachers feeding the masses the manifested kernels of Spirit. The energy helps to shift mass consciousness reality into a different direction of feeling, seeing, and interpreting things.

Vanilla is a tropical vine with a white trumpet flower that humming birds love. The oil has a very subtle and gentle quality. It helps people that lived during Lumerian times recall aspects of themselves. The Lumerian people had a gentle nature and an affinity with the Earth's elements and were more deeply connected to Earth essence than the Atlantean people. Vanilla's essence triggers memories in people who lived lifetimes as Polynesians or Tahitians. The Vanilla vine is native to Central America and also helps recall Aztec and Mayan memories.

Using the oil for transformation

Use Vanilla oil on the neck and throat to open the energy for self-expression. Inhaling Vanilla oil will help alleviate food cravings. Massage into the stomach, large and small intestine meridians to release constriction and to train energy to be absorbed in the throat chakra.

Precautions

This oil is fairly non-irritating; to be certain check for a reaction. Use 15-30 drops in 2 ounces of a base oil.

VETIVER   *Vetiveria zizanioides / andropogon – Muiricatus*
Transformations

Key: Grounds and Attunes to Earth. Helps resolve the love/hate relationship with the physical body. Develops an appreciation of nature and establishes a connection with Nature Spirits.

Growth and healing issues

Acknowledging and embracing the issues underlying sorrow, depression, terror, grief, and abandonment helps dissolve the dense energy they produce. The joy of living life in the moment is realized. Not being connected to the Earth contributes depression and in extreme cases, causes a feeling of being disconnected from life, which can lead to suicidal feelings. Feeling Earth's heartbeat forges a greater bond with life and permits dancing with the realms of Nature.

Energetic influences on the bodies and chakras

The heart awakens to Nature and aligns its energy with the root chakra to ground the energy into the physical, restoring a zest for life.

Energetics of the oil

Vetiver's energy feels like being cradled in Mother Earth's arms. Its scent recalls the Earthy smell of decaying leaves. Decay is necessary in the grand cycle of life, as it is instrumental in creating new matter from which life may emerge. Vetiver oil grounds the physical body's energy, creating a feeling of security while walking on this Earth plane. The unique dynamic of Vetiver's energy helps you to feel joyfully uplifted but at the same time grounded. The energetics of Vetiver oil connect the heart with Nature's sacred rhythmic cycles.

Vetiver oil provides a safe and nurturing energy that helps to surface feelings of abandonment and self-hatred of the physical form. The energetics awaken suppressed feelings of depression and dense thought patterns, which can be anything that is not of the love vibration and needs to be aligned with joy. Beliefs associated with restrictive thought patterns are realized and then can be changed. Creating a closer alignment with joy and happiness transforms the emotions, letting you feel the heaviness and bring it up into the heart's light. Achieving this transformation comes by giving the personality permission to accept and love whatever the issue is without judging it to be right or wrong, accepting and allowing the responses of the experience as just that—an experience.

Energetically, Vetiver supports feeling joy in this third dimensional density. It is beneficial to people who do not like being in their bodies or who have suicidal feelings. It is also a helpful energy for alienated people who feel they do not belong on this planet. Vetiver energy encourages a more joyful experience of the Earth plane. It helps develop an appreciation of Nature, enabling a deeper connection to Gaia.

Meditating with Vetiver oil helps connect you with the energy of Nature Spirits. The oil helps you attune to the energies of Elves, Fairies, Wood Nymphs, and Gnomes. A greater attunement with Nature develops, which promotes feelings of harmony and peace.

Vetiver oil comes from the root of a tropical and subtropical grass. This grass is a close cousin to Lemon Grass and Citronella. The grass needs to be two years old for the root to produce its strong scent. Vetiver awakens memories of lives lived on tropical islands and in Indonesia.

Using the oil for transformation

Vetiver feels wonderful when massaged on the soles of the feet. This supports grounding the physical form. Massaging the oil on the pubic bone and on the sacrum helps open the root chakra energy. Inhaling Vetiver oil expands the root chakra energy. A symptom of a closed root chakra is a difficulty distinguishing odors. An extreme symptom of a closed first chakra is suicidal feelings. Suicidal feelings come from the inability to connect with life. Deeply inhaling the oil while visualizing your feet growing roots into the Earth helps to ground the body and strengthens the Earth connection. Using Vetiver oil on the conception meridian helps overcome the fears of being on the Earth plane. Massaging the oil on the kidney meridian helps you live in the moment. Opening the gallbladder meridians allows life to flow unrestricted. Using the oil on the stomach meridian encourages bonding to the Earth element within.

Precautions

Be suspicious of this oil's purity because it is often diluted with synthetics or less expensive constituents. This oil is fairly non-irritating, to be certain check for a reaction. Use 15-30 drops in 2 ounces of a base oil. Overuse of this oil can cause headaches.

| *WINTERGREEN* | *Gaultheria procumbens – Ericaceae* |

Transformations

Key: Relaxes the Need to Be Logical. A desire for introspection is generated. Wisdom is perceived through interpretation of abstract symbols that stimulate knowing. The breath opens to nourish self and increases self-love and self-forgiveness.

Growth and healing issues

Relaxation transforms the mental body's rigid resistance to change. Introspection produces insight into the root causes hindering integrity and self-sufficiency. Aligning heartfelt emotions with logical thoughts diminishes the resistance to feeling love. Expanding heart energy allows for emotions to be better expressed through the physical.

Energetic influences on the bodies and chakras

Warm and soothing energy gives relief to the physical body's aches and pains. Introspection generates insights into the physical, emotional, and mental issues causing the ailments of sinusitis, arthritis, and headaches. Tension and stress caused by the bombardment of astral plane energy is released from the physical body.

Energetics of the oil

Wintergreen energy feels similar to taking a deep breath of snow-laden air, so cool and refreshing. This oil relaxes the mental body's rigid need to think logically. It aligns the mental body with the emotional body's heart energy.

The energetics of Wintergreen oil promote self-reflection for insights to actualize integrity and self-sufficiency. Wintergreen heightens the wisdom that comes from intuition and knowing. The scent stimulates the mind's ability to understand abstract thought. This knowledge easily grounds into the physical because Wintergreen's energy relaxes the mental body's resistance to change and new information.

On the physical level, Wintergreen provides relief for arthritis sufferers. Resistance to feeling love causes arthritic conditions in some people. Love is the one thing so desired in life and yet so difficult to accept. A factor complicating the ability to feel love is searching for it outside of self. You cannot find it there because it can only be found within. Working with Wintergreen oil expands the heart, enabling a greater depth of emotion to be felt and physically expressed.

Use of Wintergreen oil helps relieve tension in the physical body. This is a good oil to use for relieving headaches, especially the intense kind that feel like a collision of spirit and matter. Wintergreen oil has a very cooling effect on intense emotions. Wintergreen also soothes sore muscles created from the constant bombardment of the astral plane on the physical body. Inhaling the oils opens the sinus passages, allowing the breath to nourish all the body organs. This nourishment allows a person to feel a greater sense of self-love and self-nurturing.

Wintergreen is a species of evergreen flowering shrub. It is native to the northern United States and Canada. The bright red berries produce its aroma. Native Americans used different parts of the Wintergreen shrub for medicinal remedies.

Using the oil for transformation

Using Wintergreen on sore muscles warms and soothes them. Dilute in a carrier oil or its heating properties will be overwhelming. Submerging the body into a warm Wintergreen oil bath creates a wonderful soothing and stimulating feeling. Massaging the oil onto the temples and brow and on the liver meridian helps to alleviate headaches. Inhaling the oil opens the sinuses.

The heart responds well to Wintergreen oil; rub it into the heart area or on the heart meridian. Wintergreen's warming properties comfort the heart, enabling feelings of security and protection. Massaging the oil into the pericardium meridian amplifies the ability to love. Use the oil on the gallbladder meridian to release arthritic stiffness and hip pain. Massage joints that feel stiff with the oil to lessen the pain.

Precautions

Do not use this oil on children or infants. This essential oil can be internally toxic and potentially lethal. Be suspicious of this oil's purity because it is often diluted with synthetics or less expensive constituents. This oil can irritate the skin and mucous membranes. Dilute 1-10 drops in 2 ounces of a base oil and check for a reaction. Use only 1-5 drops in a bath. Wintergreen oil reduces the effectiveness of homeopathic remedies.

WISTERIA   *Wisteria sinensis*
Transformations

Key: Experience the Joy of Doing. Information from the Higher Self is welcomed into the heart instead of the mind. Consciousness expands to include the possibility of parallel dimensions.

Growth and healing issues

The desire to experience more joy increases. Realizing that constant busy-work is a rationalization for not making time for self-discovery leads to attaining inner stillness, and diminishes dense energies maintaining the time-space reality. Wisteria energy helps overcome feelings of possessiveness, jealousy, and pessimism.

Energetic influences on the bodies and chakras

The mind and the crown chakra are aligned, enabling them to receive and assimilate a greater amount of energy. The physical body's template is purified when it interfaces with the etheric. Higher frequency energies are grounded into the physical.

Energetics of the oil

Wisteria flowers have a wonderful sweetness that generates joyful feelings. Whatever task you are performing, Wisteria energy promotes the feeling of doing it in a true vibration of joy. Wisteria oil calms the need to stay busy. Often this busyness is an escape from attaining an inner stillness.

Wisteria oil's energy allows discovering what joy feels like on a very gentle and subtle level. This is a good oil for people who close their hearts at the mention of joy. Often these people spend a lot of time in their head. Energetically, Wisteria oil helps the mental body receive and accept information channeled through the crown chakra. The information coming through this connection enriches the meaning and enjoyment of life's many-faceted experiences. This expanded consciousness allows accepting the possibility of parallel dimensions.

Wisteria energy has an intertwining, multifaceted quality. It purifies the interface of the etheric body and the physical body. This allows the physical body to ground higher frequency energies. The crown chakra then engages the energy to align with the oneness of all things. This alignment lifts the energies of pessimism, possessiveness, and jealousy, which are passions that bind the energy into this density of time and space.

Memories of Oriental life times have a tendency to surface. Wisteria oil stimulates memories associated with grace and beauty, and helps to arouse those inner qualities.

Using the oil for transformation

Using wisteria oil on the crown chakra and base of the skull stimulates memory. Placing it behind the ears and neck also creates a feeling of joyful lightness. Use the oil on the kidney meridian to feel more joy in life. Rub the oil into a point midway down the inside calf muscle to calm stress from overachieving. Using the oil on the kidney meridian promotes self-forgiveness and helps one to live in the moment. Allow the energy of things to come and go more easily by using the oil on the lung meridian, releasing anxiety and the fear of failure. Using Wisteria oil on the percardium meridian allows the personality to relax, making it easier to feel free and open. Wisteria oil on the liver meridian balances drive and motivation.

Precautions

This oil is fairly non-irritating, to be certain check for a reaction. Use 15-30 drops in 2 ounces of a base oil. Be suspicious of this oil's purity because it is often diluted with synthetics or less expensive constituents.

YLANG-YLANG   *Cananga odorata – Anonaceae*

Transformations

Key: Calms Nerves and Integrates Emotions. Greater intimacy is felt when rejection and abandonment are embraced. Awareness of boundaries determines the appropriate use of energy. Relaxation of the mind promotes a shift in perspectives.

Growth and healing issues

Emotionally charged states dissipate. Feeling more lovable is possible when passions of anger and frustration calm. Mental concerns relax, producing insights into the root causes of fears.

Energetic influences on the bodies and chakras

Emotions integrate, clearing the emotional, mental, and etheric bodies. The electromagnetic body is revitalized for manifesting healing energy. Assimilating more healing energy calms the nervous system. The mind and physical body experience a very profound feeling of sedation and relaxation.

Energetics of the oil

Ylang-Ylang feels like a colorful, exotic, blooming flower garden where the many fragrances blending into one. Ylang-Ylang oil integrates the emotions and soothes the nervous system.

Calming the nervous system revitalizes the electromagnetic body to manifest greater amounts of healing energy. Energetically, this calms the passions of anger and frustration almost immediately in the emotional, mental, and etheric bodies. Its sedating effect produces a deeper feeling of relaxation. Ylang-Ylang is a good oil for insomniacs, because of its effectiveness in calming and soothing all the bodies.

Ylang-Ylang addresses the fear of intimacy, especially if the fear was created by an experience of rejection. Ylang-Ylang calms the passions of jealousy by generating the ability to feel more lovable. Meditation with Ylang-Ylang teaches and maintains an understanding of boundaries. This creates a sense of capability and promotes taking charge of one's power and destiny, allowing healthier relationships to form. Emotionally charged states are released by the calming effect of Ylang-Ylang. Relaxing the mind allows a change of perspective to clearly see and feel where the fear originates. Acknowledging the root cause of a fear helps to stop it from becoming a reaction and promotes feelings of choice to act rather than re-act.

Using the oil for transformation

A bath with Ylang-Ylang is a wonderful calming experience that promotes the Soul-search into your essence. Overuse of Ylang-Ylang oil could produce a headache when you are in a state of resistance. Ask an Angel for assistance in releasing this state of resistance. Once out of this state it is easier to learn to flow into the state of Divine surrender.

To overcome the fear of intimacy, use Ylang-Ylang oil on the pericardium meridian. When the triple warmer is massaged with the oil it helps establish new relationship patterns, and develops warmer heartfelt feelings. Using Ylang-Ylang on the liver meridian releases feelings of anger, frustration and sexual frigidity. Ylang-Ylang on the governing meridian calms the nervous system and helps overcome insomnia. Holding the forehead point above the bridge of the nose also relieves insomnia.

Precautions

Be suspicious of this oil's purity because it is often diluted with synthetics or less expensive constituents. This oil is fairly non-irritating, to be certain check for a reaction. Use 15-30 drops in 2 ounces of a base oil.

Glossary

AKASHIC RECORDS — Cosmic records of all time and dimensions, containing an individual's deeds, thoughts, and experiences, from past, present, and future incarnations on Earth.

ANDROGYNY — The male and female energies integrated.

ANGELIC ASPECTS — The Soul's Angelic essence.

AROMATHERAPY — A type of therapy that uses essential oils to promote physical, emotional, mental, and spiritual healing.

ASCENDED MASTERS — Beings of Light that have Ascended into another dimension and help Humanity evolve Spiritually.

ASTRAL BODY — One of the subtle bodies that surrounds the physical body and encompasses the mental and emotional auric fields.

ASTRAL PROJECTION — Also known as an out-of-the body experience. This often happens in an expanded state of reality or during sleep when the astral body separates from the physical body.

AURA — The electromagnetic energy emanating as a halo around the physical body of all life forms. The radiating energy varies in size, color, and density. It is often invisible but some psychic individuals and most animals can perceive it by sight, feeling, or hearing.

AURIC FIELD — The light vibrating around the physical body that displays the emotional, mental, and physical states.

BEINGS OF LIGHT — Energies of consciousness from the unseen realm of Angels, Ascended Masters, Devic Beings, and Nature Spirits, etc., that serve Humanity as guides and helpers on the journey.

BLUEPRINT — The consciousness that retains the third dimension. It is the perfect plan of health that the body created before entering this realm.

BODY — Vehicle that contains consciousness.

CELLULAR MEMORY — Information in the cellular conscious of the physical body imprinted by emotional and mental experiences.

CHAKRA — An energy vortex just outside of, but connected to, the physical body.

CHAKRA SYSTEM — Spiritual energy centers that connect and channel energy into the physical body. There are also many chakras outside of the body connecting to planetary energy.

CHRIST — The completed integration of the personality and Soul consciousness of Earth experiences.

CLAIRAUDIENCE — The ability to hear auditory messages and sounds from the Soul, other dimensions, and Light Beings.

CLAIRVOYANCE — The ability to perceive visual information from other dimensions, dreams, and guides pertaining to events from the past, present, and future.

COLLAPSING TIME — The ability to perceive the past, present, and future as Now.

COLLECTIVE CONSCIOUSNESS — The combined feelings, thoughts, and beliefs of groups of people, and the vibrational frequency created by it.

CONSCIOUSNESS — The awareness of knowing that is transmitted from all planes of existence.

CONSCIOUS MIND — The Ego and personality influence that directs and analysis the material based activities of life on the Earth plane.

CONSENTUAL REALITY — The agreement we make that creates and maintains this third dimension existence.

CREATIVE VISUALIZATION — Using the mind to imagine and manifest mental images and feelings.

CROWN CHAKRA — The seventh chakra that symbolizes enlightenment.

DENSITY — Heavy-feeling consciousness, which originates from low frequency vibration containing fear, anger, anxiety, and other thoughts, emotions, or experiences that resonate with the third dimension.

DEVAS (NATURE SPIRITS) — Souls associated with various forms of nature that exist on a different frequency and dimension than the physical plane. They are the Angels of the plant, animal, and mineral kingdoms.

DIMENSIONS — Different planes of reality that sustain life in a variety of forms and consciousness.

DISCERNMENT — The ability to Intuitively know without judgment.

DIVINE RIGHT USE OF EMPATHING — The ability to sense intuitive information through the body in an appropriate manner that does not own or attach to the information personally.

DIVINE RIGHT TIMING — The ability to spiritually evolve in the correct manner and process.

DUALITY — The state of separation from Spirit. The polarity of consciousness that separates the world into black and white, good and evil, etc.

EGO — The consciousness that considers itself to be a separate Self. It believes itself to be in control of life. It reinforces the state of separation and self-limitation and maintains the third dimension reality and karma.

ELEMENTALS — Beings of Light that are the energies of manifestation, fire, water, air, earth, wood, etc.

EMBRACING — totally loving an action, belief, situation, etc. Once the energy is totally loved—embraced into the heart—it is transmuted into another form.

EMOTION — Internal feelings generated by the emotional body's reaction to experiences. These feelings are expressed as attitudes and as sensations in the physical body. In the mental body emotions are expressed as beliefs and attitudes.

EMOTIONAL BODY — A subtle body and vehicle of consciousness that records the emotional attitudes, beliefs, thoughts, and experiences from the past, present, and future.

EMPATHING — The ability to deeply feel and sympathize with what another person is feeling. Sensing these perceptions through the physical, emotional, and mental bodies, the receiver often believes them as theirs own.

ENCODEMENTS — Consciousness embedded into the Unconscious mind and often dormant.

ENERGY FREQUENCIES —The programmed consciousness from the essence
of all existence that creates vibrational rhythms.

ESSENTIAL OILS —The distilled oil of a plant; the plant's lifeblood. Oils are
imprinted with Devic consciousness that influences responses in
Humanity. An oil is the signature of the plant and enables communication
with Spirit.

ETHERIC — Refers to the vibratory emanations of all life on the earth and
other dimensions.

ETHERIC BODY — A vehicle for subtle body energy that emanates outside of
the physical body encompassing the mental, emotional and auric bodies.

ETHERIC TEMPLATES —The blueprint replica of the physical body.

ETHERS — Emanating energy that connects all existence and is faster than
the speed of light.

FEAR — All that which is not light and maintains the reality of separateness
from Spirit.

FRAGMENTED SELF — Parts of the ego and personality that dissociate, creating internal conflict.

GAIA —The name for the sentimental being known as Earth or Terra, the
great Mother of all.

GRACE —The Divine force that is available on the planet to activate individ-
ually or collectively in order for transmutation, transcendence, and transformation to occur. This energy is the spiritual aspect of forgiveness that
generates the ability to become more compassionate and accepting.

GROUNDED ASCENSION —The process of anchoring the Soul consciousness
in the physical body. Enabling the physical body to transform into the
light body.

GROUP CONSCIOUSNESS —The collective consciousness of a group or community of people.

HIGHER SELF —The self that is a vehicle to impart Soul knowledge into the
personality or ego. This self has all information from past, present, and
future lives and imparts cosmic consciousness to the physical.

Inner Child — The being within that often shuts down in childhood, creating beliefs that stimulate reactionary patterns.

Intent — The purpose and drive and focus to obtain what you desire.

Inner Guides — Beings of Light that relate in a manner that expands our awareness and encourages growth.

Inner Self — The intuitive part of us that knows our Divine self.

Integrity — The manner in which we express our Divinity through our actions in relating to the world. Integrity arises from the integration of Soul energy with the personality.

Intuition — The ability to know through feeling, hearing, or seeing the messages imparted through the Higher Self, Guides, Angels, etc. This awareness is perceived as subtle energy vibrations, interpreting the language of life.

Imprint — All the thought forms containing the personality's experiences and the Soul's knowledge of true Spiritual existence.

Judgment — A process of filtering the perceptions of the emotional and mental body that analyzes what we see, hear, and feel. This separation and labeling of experiences maintains the state of duality and limitation.

Karma — The cause and effects of all actions through all life times. A force or action that insures balance by taking responsibility for obligations incurred from previous experiences.

Kundalini — A powerful spiritual energy that lies dormant in the base of the physical spine. Once awakened, spiritual growth results.

Knowing — Awareness that does not need validation. Accessing imprinted Soul wisdom.

Light Beings — Spirit Guides, Individual Souls, Ascended Masters, Entities, Angels, Extraterrestrial, and others that exist as the Unseen Realm in other dimensions. They assist Humanity on the Earth Plane.

Light Body — The expanded vibrational frequency of consciousness that exists in the etheric and is connected to the Soul.

Linear Time — Mechanical time that is qualifies time as past, present, and future.

LOWER SELF — The total of the subtle etheric bodies and the physical body.

MASS CONSCIOUSNESS — The collective consciousness that limits the definition of reality to the physical and is accepted by the majority of people as truth.

MASTER — A Being of Light that has obtained the "Christ Consciousness" and is able to transcend the limitation of time and space, as well as being able to materialize and dematerialize.

MENTAL BODY — A subtle body that records all thoughts, patterns, and beliefs generated from past, present and future experiences. The linear process that the personality uses to understand reality through the facilities of the rational, logical, intuitive, and intellectual minds.

MEDITATION — An inward reflection and contemplation on self or nature; quiet time that promotes the connection to Source, thoughts, or beliefs that provide answers to what one is seeking.

MERIDIANS — Energy channels that carry the physical body's life force connecting into specific organs. There are many additional spiritual meridians not yet activated in the physical body.

MULTI-DIMENSIONALITY — The ability to simultaneously perceive different energy vibrations and planes of existence in a non-linear fashion.

MULTI-SENSORY — Ability to perceive information through many channels at once.

MUSCLE TESTING — A process for accessing information from the unconscious.

NLP — Neuro-Linguistic Programming. Neuro refers to the mind and nervous system through which external information is received into the physical. Linguistic refers to the language of the mind, how it interprets the world through the senses, for example—auditory, visual, kinesthetic, olfactory, and gustatory. Programming refers to the patterns created by reactions to a stimulus.

NOW — Being in the moment of time.

ONENESS —The all-inclusive reality of "All That There Is," which is the all-knowing knowledge. Its alternate names are Super-consciousness, the I Am Presence, or Christ Consciousness.

PARALLEL LIVES — Experiences that are occurring simultaneous to our current consciousness. We are often not aware of them. These lives are created by possibilities set in motion through the choices we make and experiences needed to fulfill Spiritual purpose in some way. As we become more multidimensional we will have "bleed-through" of these lives and comprehension of the parts of the Self living in them.

PAST LIVES —The experiences of various lifetimes previous to this present life as measured in linear time. In actuality they are occurring Now. These experiences provide accessible resources and talents to draw upon in this reality. They also can provide keys that illuminate the root-cause of an issue. Past life regression is a method of increasing our ability to accept multidimensionality.

PENDULUM — A small crystal, paper clip, or any small object attached to a string. Its purpose is to diagnose, divine, or analyze information.

PERCEPTION — How we synthesize and order reality.

PHYSICAL BODY —The vehicle of consciousness that maintains the third dimension reality.

POLARITY —The separation of energy into positive and negative charges creating the state of duality.

PRANA — A term to describe the Divine breath which is the life force energy that sustains and nourishes the physical body.

REALM — A dimension of reality.

REALITY — Our collective manifestations of existence. There are many realities.

RESISTANCE — A survival or defense that the emotional, mental, and physical bodies engage to protect the self by self-limitation.

SELF —The personality created through experiences of the emotional, mental, and physical bodies. We have many fragmented selves and the journey home requires embracing them into wholeness. Usually this self is denoted in small case letters. Capitalized Self refers to the Soul or spiritual Self and is also known as the Higher-Self.

SEPARATION — The state of exclusion from Source or Spirit and Self.

SIGNATURE — The individual vibration of a person, place or thing.

SOLAR PLEXUS CHAKRA — The 4th chakra, center of the will.

SOUL — An individualized aspect of the universal Divine essence.

SOUL BODY — An etheric subtle body that vibrates around the etheric body. It records all incarnations and is connected to a soul group that may or may not be incarnate at the present.

SOUL LIGHT — The amount of energy emanating from the Soul or Spirit.

SOURCE — The Light of all creation containing the knowing of Oneness. It emanates information through the Higher Self for the personality self to interpret.

SPIRIT — The origin of spiritual, cosmic knowing from which all information and creation emanates. This is the I Am Presence.

SPIRITUAL BODY — The body directly connected to cosmic consciousness of the Godhead; the I Am Presence.

SPIRITUALITY — The journey back to Source that comes from learning to totally love and accept self without judgment.

SUBTLE BODIES — All the bodies surrounding and existing outside of the physical body.

TELEPATHY — Transmission of thoughts that communicate with people, animals, plants, and Beings from other dimensions. This communication is perceived in the mind through methods other than the five physical senses.

TEMPLATES — The blueprint that records the knowledge of Spiritual perfection.

THIRD DIMENSION — The reality we live in, recognized as tangible and constrained by the laws of time and space.

THIRD EYE CHAKRA — The sixth chakra, center of visualization and conception of knowledge.

Time / Space Continuum — The organization of time as past, present and future occurring NOW.

Thought Forms — Densities, shapes, or forms that are a consequence of thoughts from the mind, emotions, and collective consciousness.

Unconscious Mind — The all-knowing part of the physical mind that records and contains all information of past, present, and future experiences from the emotional, mental, physical bodies. It is outside our conscious awareness. Links between the subtle bodies and the unconscious mind can be developed to guide the conscious mind to Source and Spirit.

Universal Mind — The collective consciousness of all that has been experienced and is available to be accessed through connection with Spirit or Source.

Unseen Realm — Life beyond the third dimension.

Vibration — The energy patterns emitted from all life, substance, and the ethers moving in cyclic wave frequencies of energy. On Earth's three-dimensional plane, vibration is manifested as sound, color, light, and form.

Yin / Yang — The balance of opposites, such as male/female and receiving/projecting, that are part of the polarity consciousness.

Wave Patterns — The vibrational frequencies of the ethers that influence the creation of all manifestation.

Bibliography

ACUPRESSURE, REFLEXOLOGY, AND MASSAGE

Beck, Mark, *The Theory and Practice of Therapeutic Massage*. New York: Milady Publishing, 1988.

Blate, Michael, *The Natural Healer's Acupressure Handbook: G-JO Fingertip Technique*. Florida: Falkynor, 1976.

Cerney, J.V., *Acupressure: Acupuncture Without Needles*. New York: Simon and Schuster, 1974.

Gach, Michael Reed, *Acupressure's Potent Points*. New York: Bantam Books, 1990.

Haas, E., *Staying Healthy with the Seasons*. Millbrae, CA: 1980.

Hin, Kuan, *Chinese Massage and Acupressure*. New York: Bergh Publishing Inc., 1991.

Houston, F.M., *The Healing Benefits of Acupressure*. Connecticut: Keats Publishing, Inc., 1991.

Mole, Peter, *Acupuncture: Energy Balancing for Body, Mind, and Spirit*. Massachusetts: Element, Inc., 1992.

Segal, Maybelle, *Reflexology*. California: Wilshire Book Company,, 1976.

Whisenant, William, Ph.D., *Psychological Kinesiology: Changing the Body's Beliefs*. Texas: Monarch Butterfly Productions, 1990.

Raheem, Aminah, Ph.D., *Soul Return: Integrating Body, Psyche, and Spirit*. California: Aslan Publishing, 1991.

Smith, Fritz Fredrick, M.D., *Inner Bridges*. Georgia: Humanics New Age, 1994.

AROMATHERAPY

Cunnighan, Scott, *Magical Aromatherapy*. Minnesota: Llewellyn Publications, 1990.

Davis, Patricia, *Aromatherapy: An A-Z*. London: C.W. Daniel Company, 1988.

Greer, Mary, *The Essence of Magic*. California: New Castle Publishing, 1993.

Jackson, Judith, *Scentual Touch*. New York: Fawcett Columbine, 1987.

Junemann, Monika, *Enchanting Scents*. Wisconsin: Lotus Light, 1988.

Keller, Erich, *Complete Home Guide to Aromatherapy*. California: H. J. Kramer, 1991.

Lavabre, Marcel, *Aromatherapy Workbook*. Vermont: Healing Arts Press, 1990.

Lawless, Julia, *The Encyclopedia of Essential Oils*. Massachusetts: Element Inc., 1992.

Ryman, Daniele, *Aromatherapy: The Complete Guide to Plant and Flower Essences for Health and Beauty*. New York: Batman Books, 1993.

Tisserand, Robert, *The Art of Aromatherapy*. Vermont: Destiny Books, 1977.

Valnet, Jean, M.D., *The Practice of Aromatherapy*. Vermont: Healing Arts Press, 1990.

BOTANICAL REFERENCES

Hoffmann, David, *The Holistic Herbal*. Scotland: The Findhorn Press, 1985.

Jensen, Bernard, D.C., Ph.D., *Herbal Handbook*. California: Bernard Jensen, Publishing, 1988.

Kloss, Jethro, *Back to Eden*. California: Woodbridge Press, 1971.

Lepore, Donald N.D., *The Ultimate Healing System*. Utah: Woodland Books, 1988.

Rose, Jeanne, *Herbs and Things*. New York: Perigee Books, 1983.

Rose, Jeanne, *Modern Herbal*. New York: Perigee Books, 1987.

Tierra, Michael, *The Way of Herbs*. New York: Pocket Books, 1983.

Tompkins, Peter, and Christopher Bird, *Secrets of The Soil*. New York: Harper and Row, 1989.

Stuart, Malcom, *Encyclopedia of Herbs and Herbalism*. New York: Crescent Books, 1981.

ENERGY, AURAS, CHAKRAS AND SUBTLE BODIES

Besant, Annie, *A Study in Consciousness*. Illinois: The Theosophical Publishing House, 1975.

Brennan, Barbara Ann, *Hands of Light*. New York: Bantam Books, 1987.

Carrington Hereward and Sylvan Muldoon, *The Projection of the Astral Body*. Maine: Samuel Weiser, Inc., 1984.

Colton, Ann Ree, *Kundalini Wes*. California: ARC Publishing Company,, 1978.

Cousens, Gabriel M.D., *Spiritual Nutrition and The Rainbow Diet*. Company,, Cassandra Press, 1986.

Chia, Mantak, *Awaken Healing Energy through the Tao*. New York: 1983.

Gimble, Theo, *Healing through Colour*. London: C.W. Daniel Company, Ltd., 1980

Leadbetter, C.W., *The Chakras*. Illinois: The Theosophical Pub House, 1972.

Lansdowne, Zachary, *The Chakras and Esoteric Healing*. Maine: Samuel Weiser, 1986.

Jafolla, Richard, *Soul Surgery: The Ultimate Self-Healing*. California: DeVorss and Company,, 1987.

Judith, Anodea, *Wheels of Life*. Minnesota: Llewellyn Publishing, 1987

Kuthumi, (Mark L. Prophet), *Studies of the Human Aura*. California: Summit University. Press, 1971.

Tansley, David, Chakras, *Rays and Radionics*. London: C.W. Daniel Company,, 1984.

Schwarz, Jack, *The Human Energy Systems*. New York: Dutton, 1980

Sui, Choa Kok, *Pranic Healing*. Maine: Samuel Weiser, 1990.

Powell, A.E., *The Astral Body*. Illinois: The Theosophical Publishing, House, 1972.

Powell, A.E., *The Etheric Double*. Illinois: The Theosophical Publishing, House, 1969.

Pierrakos, John C., *The Core Energetic Process*. New York: Institute for the
    New Age, 1975

Zukaw, Gary, *The Dancing Wu Li Masters: An Overview of the New Physics*. New
    York: William Morrow and Company,, 1979

_____, *The Seat of the Soul*. New York: William Morrow and Company,, 1979

MIND AND BODY HEALING

Bandler, Richard, *Using Your Brain — For A Change*. Utah: Real People Press,
    1979.

Bandler, Richard, and Grinder, John, *Frogs Into Princes*. Utah: Real People
    Press, 1979.

Borysenko, Joan Ph.D., *Minding the Body, Mending the Mind*. New York:
    Bantam Books, 1987.

Erickson, Milton H., M.D., and Rossi, Ernest, *Hypnotic Realities*. New York:
    Irvington Publishing, 1976.

Gawain, Shakti, *Creative Visualization*. California: Whatever Publishing, 1978.

Griscom, Chris, *The Healing of Emotion*. New York: Simon and Schuster,
    1988.

Hay, Louise, *Heal Your Body*. California: Hay House, Inc., 1982.

James, Tad, and Woodsmall, Wyatt, *Time Line and The Basis of Personality*.
    California: Meta Publishing, 1988.

Liese, Bruce, Cory Newman, Fred Wright, and Aaron Beck, *Cognitive Therapy
    of Substance Abuse*. New York: Guilford Press, 1993.

Keyes, Ken, *Handbook to Higher Consciousness*. Kentucky: Living Love Center,
    1975.

Lowen, Alexander, M.D., *The Betrayal of the Body*. New York: Collier Books,
    1967.

Monroe, Robert A., *Journeys Out of the Body*. New York: Anchor Press, 1977.

Pullar, Philippa, and Lilla Bek, *The Seven Levels of Healing*. Australia: Century
    Hutchinson Publishing Group, 1986.

Reich, Wilhelm, *Character Analysis*. London, Vision Press, 1950.

Sherwood, Keith, *The Art of Spiritual Healing*. Minnesota: Llewellyn
    Publishing, 1986.

Upledger, John, *Your Inner Physician and You*. California: North Atlantic
    Books, 1991.

Wilson, Robert Anton, *Quantum Psychology*. Arizona: New Falcon Publishing,
    1990.

METAPHYSICS

Alper, Frank, *Universal Law*. California: Quantum Productions, 1986.

Bailey, Alice A., *Esoteric Healing*. New York: Lucis Publishing, Company,,
    1980.

———, *Esoteric Psychology, Vol. I,* New York: Lucis Publishing Company,, 1975

———, *Esoteric Psychology, Vol. II*. New York: Lucis Publishing, Company,,
    1975.

———, *Ponder on This*. New York: Lucis Publishing, Company,, 1980

———, *Initiation, Human and Solar*. New York: Lucis Publishing, Company,,
    1967

———, *Telepathy and the Etheric Vehicle*. New York: Lucis Publishing,
    Company,,

Blavastsky, Helena, *The Secret Doctrine*. Illinois: The Theosophical Publishing
    House, 1980.

Carey Ken, *Vision*. Michigan: UNI*SUN, 1985.

———, *Starseed Transmissions*. Michigan: UNI*SUN, 1985.

Colton, Ann Ree, *Watch Your Dreams*. California: ARC Publishing Company,
    1973.

———, *Islands of Dreams*. California: California: ARC Publishing Company

———, *Ethical ESP*. California: ARC Publishing Company, ___

———, *Men in White Apparel*. California: ARC Publishing Company, ___

———, *The Human Spirit*. California: ARC Publishing Company, ___

Erbe, Peter, *God I AM: From Tragic to Magic*. Australia, TRIAD Publishing,
    1991.

Haigh, John, *Serving Planet Earth*. Australia: Sontar Communications, 1981.

Levi, *The Aquarian Gospel of Jesus the Christ*. California: Devorss and
     Company, 1982.

May, Robert M., *Physicians of the Soul*. Massachusetts: Element, Inc., 1991.

Montgomery, Ruth, *The World Before*. New York: Fawcett Crest Book, 1977.

Prophet, Mark L., *Kuthumi Studies of the Human Aura*. California: Summit
     University Press, 1971.

Spangler, David, *The Laws of Manifestation*. California: Findhorn Foundation,
     1978.

MYTHS AND HISTORY

Campbell, Joseph, *The Hero with a Thousand Faces*. New Jersey: Princeton
     University Press, 1949.

_____, *The Mythic Image*. New Jersey: Princeton University Press, 1974.

Lehner, Mark, *The Egyptian Heritage*. Virginia Beach: A.R.E. Press, 1983.

Walker, Barbara, *The Woman's Dictionary of Symbols and Sacred Objects*. New
     York: Harper and Row, 1988.

ANGELS, NATURE SPIRITS, AND LIGHT BEINGS

Andrews, Ted, *Enchantment of the Faerie Realm*. Minnesota: Llewellyn
     Publishing, 1993.

_____, *Animals Speak*. Minnesota: Llewellyn Publishing, 1993.

Arquelles, Jose, *Surfers of the Zuvuya*. New Mexico: Bear and Company,
     1988.

_____, *Earth Ascending*, New Mexico: Bear and Company, 1984.

Azena, St. Germain, *Earth Birth Changes*. Australia: TRIAD Publishing, 1993.

Briggs, Katharine, *An Encyclopedia of Fairies*. New York: Pantheon Books,
     1976.

Essene, Virginia, and Ann Valentin, *Cosmic Revelation*. California: Spiritual
     Education Endeavors, 1987.

Findhorn Community, *The Findhorn Garden.* New York: Harper and Row Publishing, 1976.

Hall, Manly P., *Unseen Forces.* Illinois: The Theosophical Publishing House, 1978.

Hawken, Paul, *The Magic of Findhorn.* New York: Bantam Books, 1974.

King, Jani, *The P'TAAH Tapes: An Act of Faith.* Australia, TRIAD Publishing, 1991.

King, Jani, *The P'TAAH Tapes: Transformation of the Species.* TRIAD Publishing, 1991.

Maclean, Dorothy, *To Hear The Angels Sing.* Illinois: Lorian Press, 1980.

Milanovich, Norma, *We, The Archturians.* New Mexcio Athena Publishing, 1990.

Price, John, *The Super Beings.* Texas: Aranan IV Publishing, 1981.

Solara, *The Legend of Altazar.* California: Star-Borne Unlimited, 1987.

Solara, *The Star-Borne: A Rememberance for the Awakened Ones.* Arizona: Star-Borne, 1989.

Solara, *EL*AN*RA: The Healing of Orion.* Arizona: Star-Borne, 1991.

Van Gelder, Dora, *The Real World of Fairies.* Illinois: Quest Books, 1977.

Wright, Machaelle *Small, Behaving As if The God In All Life Mattered.* Vermont: Perelandra, 1987.

VIBRATIONAL HEALING

Bach, Edward, M.D. and F. J. Wheeler, M.D., *The Bach Flower Remedies.* Connecticut: Keats Health Books, 1979.

Bentof, Itzhak, *Stalking the Wild Pendulum: On the Mechanics of Consciousness.* New York: Bantam Books, 1977.

Cheney, Margaret, *Tesla: Man Out of Time.* New York: Bantam Doubleday Publishing Group, Inc., 1981

Chia, Mantak, *Awaken Healing Energy through the Tao.* New York: Aurora Press, 1983.

Cunningham, Donna, and Andrew Ramer, *Further Dimensions of Healing Addictions.* California: Cassandra Press, 1988.

David, William, *The Harmonics of Sound, Color and Vibration.* California: DeVorss and Company, 1980.

Gerber, Richard, *Vibrational Medicine.* New Mexico: Bear and Company, 1988.

Gurudas, *Flower Essences and Vibrational Healing.* New Mexico: Brotherhood of Life, Inc., 1983.

Gurudas, *The Spiritual Properties of Herbs.* California: Cassandra Press, 1988.

_____, *Gem Elixirs and Vibrational Healing, Vol. I.* California: Cassandra Press, 1985.

_____, *Gem Elixirs and Vibrational Healing, Vol. II.* California: Cassandra Press, 1986.

Hall, Manly, *Healing: Divine Art.* Los Angeles: Philosophical Research Society, Inc., 1971

Scheffer, Mechthild, *Bach Flower Therapy.* Vermont: Healing Arts Press, 1988.

Wall, Vicky, *The Miracle of Colour Healing.* London, Aquarian Press, 1990.

Wright, Machaelle Small, *Flower Essences.* Virginia: Prelandra, Ltd., 1988.

Index

A

Abandonment, feelings of, 95, 96, 123, 178

Abies alba, 116–19

Acorus calamus angustatus, 78–81

Acupressure/acupuncture, 22

Addictions, 165–67

Allergies, 51

Allspice, 54–56

Amyris (Amyris balsamifera), 57–59

Angelica Root (Angelica archangelical), 59–62

Angels, 60–61, 69–70

Anger, 98, 99, 100–101

Aniba rosaeodora, 176–80

Animals, 195

Anorexia, 115

Anxieties, 73

Apium graveolens, 93–95

Apple cider vinegar, 43

Artemisia dracunculus, 202–4

Arthritis, 214

Attraction, law of, 9

B

Baking soda, 43

Balance, maintaining, 107–8

Basil, 65–68

Baths, 17, 42–45

Bay Laurel, 135–36

Bergamot, 69–72

Betrayal, 152, 153, 154

Black Pepper, 73–75

Bladder meridian, 27–28

Bleed-through, 11–12

Bosellia carteri, 119–21

Burdens, uplifting, 81

C

Cajeput, 75–78

Calamus Root, 78–81

Camphor of Borneo, 81–84

Cananga odorata, 217–18

Candida, 206

Cardamon Seed, 84–86

Carrot Seed, 86–90

Cedar (Cedrus atlantica Manetti), 90–92

Celery Seed, 93–95

Chakras, 18–21
    defined, 18
    locations and associations, 20–21
    outside the body, 21

Chamomile (Chamaemelum nobile), 95–97

Change, 3, 198

Chaparral tea, 43

Chi, 22, 25

Childbirth, 186, 200–201

Childhood, unpleasant experiences in, 54, 55, 105, 178

Children, essential oils and, 51

Chinese medicine, traditional, 22, 32

Chlorine bleach, 43

Cinnamon (Cinnamonum zeylanicum/cassia), 98–100

Citronella, 100–102

Citrus aurantifolia, 142–43

Citrus aurantium amara, 165–67

Citrus aurantium bergamia, 69–72

Citrus aurantium bigaradia, 150–52

Citrus aurantium sinensis, 155–56

Citrus limon, 138–40

Citrus reticulata, 198–202

Citrus x paradisi, 126–28

Clairaudience, 63, 135, 136

Clairvoyance, 135, 136

Clary Sage, 102–4

Clay plaster, red, 42

Clove Bud, 104–7

Clover, red, 44

Commiphora myrrha, 146–48

Compassion, 109, 176

Conception Vessel, 22, 30–31

Conscious empowerment, 128

Consciously present, 198

Consciousness
    expanding and grounding, 86–87
    seven levels of, 128–30

Control, 193

Cosmic knowledge, 62, 63

Time
collapsing, 12
-space continuum, 11
Trance channeling, 95, 96, 137
Triple Warmer meridian, 29–30
Trust, 147
Truth
of life, 181
speaking your, 54–56

U
Unseen Realm, communication with, 69

V
Vanilla (Vanilla planifolia), 208–10
Vetiver (Vetiveria zizanioides/andropogon), 211–13
Vibrational aromatherapy, 13
Vibrational healing, 11–12
Vibrational theory, 8–10

W
Will
to live, 159
Spiritual, 133
Wintergreen, 213–15
Wisdom
ancestral, 184
of peace, 95
perception of, 213, 214

Wisteria (Wisteria sinensis), 215–17
Worry, 73

Y
Yeast conditions, 206
Yin and yang, 22, 25
Ylang-Ylang, 217–18

Z
Zingiber officinalis, 123–26

About the Author

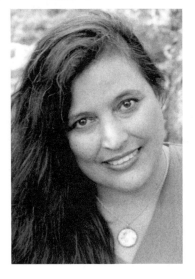

Deborah Eidson is a ten-year veteran of aromatherapy with an extensive background in botany, which she studied at the University of Texas. She is a registered massage therapist who uses craniosacral therapy and Bach Flower Remedies in her practice. Deborah is a lightworker and intuitive energetic channeler. She has extensive training in a variety of healing modalities. Her system incorporates various eclectic tools and combines them with essential oils in this unique method of Vibrational Healing.

To learn more about Deborah Eidson's consultations and other services, her schedule of upcoming events, or her energy work, visit her website at www.streamsoflight.com. To make an appointment for a private consultation, via phone or in person, e-mail spirit@streamsoflight.com, or phone (512) 462-9993, or write to Deborah at 1908-B Lightsey Road, Austin, Texas, 78704.